TO DREAM THE PERFECT ORGANIZATION

OTHER BOOKS, FILMS, TAPES BY JOEL FORT, M.D.

BOOKS

Sound Mind, Sound Society: A Positive Approach to Psychological and Social Health, University of California, Independent Study, Berkeley, 1980.

Youth: Sex, Drugs and Life. Yearbook Medical Publishers, Chicago, 1976.

American Drugstore: Alcohol to Valium. Little, Brown & Co., Boston, 1975.

Alcohol: Our Biggest Drug Problem. McGraw-Hill, New York, 1973.

The Pleasure Seekers. Bobbs Merrill, and Grove Press, New York, 1969.

FILMS

The Unreasonable Man, KQED-TV and Public Broadcasting System, San Francisco, 1969.

To Make a Start in Ending Violence, KPIX-TV, San Francisco and Psychological Films, Orange, CA, 1970.

Heroin, Bailey Film Associates, Santa Monica, CA, 1968.

TAPES

Love, Hate, Anger, and Violence, University of California Extension Media Center, Berkeley, CA, 1975.

Contemporary Issues in American Society, Behavioral Sciences Tape Library, Ft. Lee, NJ, 1967.

TO DREAM
THE PERFECT ORGANIZATION

Creating new and human organizations
Solving social and health problems
Fighting the "system"

JOEL FORT, M.D.   **LOTHAR SALIN, M.A.**

Published by Third Party Publishing Company
A division of Third Party Associates, Inc.
Oakland, California

ACKNOWLEDGEMENTS

With gratitude and respect for Meg, Helen, Van, Carolyn, Melanie, Nan, Bernie, Beth, John, Liz, Carrie, Reda, Irit, Jerry, Brigid, Linda, Mimi, and the hundreds of other staff members who spontaneously joined, shared, believed, and helped to build and maintain the Center for Solving Problems — FORT HELP; the Board of Directors, especially Owen Chamberlain, Toni Rembe, Art Lantz, and Karen Stone; and the thousands of guests who telephoned and came for help.

TO DREAM THE PERFECT ORGANIZATION

Library of Congress Catalog Number: 80-53829
International Standard Book Number: 0-89914-005-X

Printed in the United States of America

CONTENTS

CHAPTER 1

THE DREAM
AND THE DREAMERS
WHAT FORT HELP WAS TO BE

The dreamers of the day are dangerous men for they may act their dream with open eyes and make it possible. —T. E. Lawrence

THE DREAM

We are a bureaucratic, organizational society. We are born in bureaucratic hospitals and educated in bureaucratic schools. Most of us spend our work lives in highly bureaucratized institutions, involving rigid hierarchical and authoritarian structures.

Fort Help was and is different. In order to provide a new and successful approach to some of the major social and health problems of our society, we developed a rare organizational style that built in participatory democracy for our staff. Rather than structuring and ordering each aspect of a program, we encouraged individual growth and leadership. Sometimes such freedom can be difficult, but we know that ultimately we are stronger for the trying.

We fuse the individual and the organization so that both, simultaneously, obtain optimal effectiveness. We have employee-centered consensual leadership, flexible and tailored to the situation, and groupings that are more rational and humane while preserving basic human rights. We minimize organizational side effects in order to provide much satisfaction for the individual.

We intended from the beginning to replace bureaucracy with an adaptive, problem-solving system of diverse specialists and generalists, linked together by coordinating "executives" moving back and forth from management to service. We believe that a mature person learns from a "perfect organization" to cope with rapid change, live with ambiguity, identify with the adaptive process, and be self-directed. Individuals working in such a system derive their satisfaction, identity, and status from helping others and from solving problems. This was, and is still, our dream.

THE DREAMERS

Like the dreams that come at night, daydreams can be elaborate, exciting, and beset with unknown terrors. So was the making of Fort Help, the San Francisco community-based center for solving human problems. It began out of the diverse training and life experience of Dr. Joel Fort, and his search for better alternatives to bureaucracy, psychiatry, exploitation, and alienation. Lothar Salin was one of the many who were attracted to the experiment. At the time, we thought that few would note nor long remember what a small band of constructive dissenters built with their brains and hands. This is our story.

As Lothar sees him, Joel is an innovator, an idea man with well-developed ethical principles who is not concerned with the precedents and technical difficulties of his proposals. Lothar, on the other hand, prefers to take untested ideas and make them work by finding their strengths and weaknesses. He tries to anticipate the unforeseen events that may be inherent in what has taken place so far.

Joel's relationship with power is unusually complex. He considers power — the forcing of others to comply — optimally unnecessary, to be used with reluctance only in emergencies. Believing leadership to be mainly inspirational, facilitative, and educative, he is nevertheless capable of strong and decisive action. It was usually difficult for him throughout our history to hold back, to share leadership and experience staff decisions he often disagreed with. But he took charge only when forced to. Power, he believes, needs to be a presence that is consistent as well as clearly defined, but not dependent on titles, salary, publicity, threats, or bribery. In an organizational framework, the balance of power is best manifested in a system where the power of expertise is balanced against that of number. Each, if unchecked, will degenerate, as we customarily observe in coercive administration on the one hand, and workers' collectives or unions on the other.

HOW THEY MET

In April, 1970, a friend of Lothar's discovered that her 17-year-old son was mainlining heroin. Deeply shaken, she begged Lothar to find a place where her son could get treatment before being caught by the police. A counselor he trusted told him, "Look up Joel Fort, who runs the Center for Special Problems in San Francisco and is doing something to help addicts and others." He found out that the center was part of the city-county government's health department services. Upon presenting himself there and asking about the services, he was brusquely told, "Intake for new patients is in the afternoon and Dr. Fort has not been at this clinic for several years, but you can probably find him at Glide." To some of the traditional city government staff and administrators, Joel was judged an anathema for his independence and antibureaucratic actions, although he was the creator of that center in 1965.

Glide Memorial United Methodist Church, under the leadership of the Reverend Cecil Williams, had become San Francisco's house of God for the counterculture. So Lothar went to Glide Church and wound up in a small back office with an efficient, humane, and precise young woman who said he had indeed come to the right place and that she was Meg Holmberg, Dr. Fort's assistant. But Meg could not offer immediate help for Lothar's friend and her son. Joel was presently at work on plans for a new, nonbureaucratic center, but it would be some months before it would be in operation.

But this was no ordinary encounter, and Meg was soon telling Lothar that she was working with Joel Fort because she admired his work so much. Lothar was soon telling her that he was a business executive ready for a career change, that he taught classes in communication skills and did consulting work in management and organizations. Meg described both the place on Howard Street (in San Francisco) that Joel had rented for his center and the staff that he was assembling. She said Joel did not feel one had to be a trained psychotherapist in order to help people. She continued: "As a matter of fact, with your knowledge of communication and your background in organizing, you sound exactly like the kind of person he is looking for. Why don't I arrange a time when the two of you can get together — I'm sure he would be interested in meeting you!"

Lothar was taken aback because he did have an interest in the parameters of psychotherapy. He had recently submitted an application to the graduate program in social work at the University of California at Berkeley, but it had been swamped in a 200:1 application-acceptance ratio. He felt an outsider and the idea that this seemingly well-known man would want to include him on the staff of a place doing new and wonderful things in helping people sounded preposterous, to say the least. But Meg can somehow make the unreasonable sound matter-of-fact. The appointment was made, and he went, fated to become one of many to make career changes with Joel's inspiration.

Lothar arrived at the National Center for Solving Special Social and Health Problems, which occupied most of the ground floor of a former candy factory and warehouse in San Francisco's industrial area. He hadn't expected anything fancy on the outside; on the inside he was ready for informal clothes and shabby furniture. But he wasn't prepared for the shock of actually stepping into the building. He had expected the new center to be another rabbit warren mental health clinic. It wasn't just that there wasn't any furniture. The interior had yet to be built! Huge, circular, concrete pillars were holding up the structure, but the only "rooms" were a vault constructed by the previous tenants, and a restroom. Everything else was wide open space, with lumber, pillows and foam rubber pieces strewn around, electrical extension cords running here and there, and fifty people sitting, standing, or milling around.

Had he come to the wrong place?

He saw a man and a woman walk into the restroom together, which took him by surprise. He wasn't "ready" for that. And then, just as he was about to give up on the whole strange idea, two new people appeared on the scene. One carried some lumber and started measuring the distance between two columns. The other, dressed in a large-patterned suit with deeptone shirt, pointed to various corners and piles of debris. Lothar suddenly realized the man in the suit was Joel Fort and that this was indeed the place he was looking for.

HOW OTHERS BECAME A PART

Part of our book is the story of this low-rent, bare, concrete space becoming the home away from home for the many of us who came to it because we had heard something exciting about it or Joel Fort. Some were professionals in the health field looking for a less-stifling atmosphere; most were outsiders to therapy. Some were students. Some were young, and some had reached middle age. There were superhips and superstraights with a lot in the middle: housewives, ex-acidheads, former radicals, transsexuals, women's libbers, and hangers-on. Most of them were at loose ends in their personal and/or working lives and in various stages of alienation, looking for new meaning, for something to believe in, maybe an alternative to traditional "success."

Just what kind of people became part of the Fort Help staff? Where did they come from and what were they looking for? Most of them were strongly committed and altruistic, especially in the early days, when being at Fort Help took precedence over almost anything else in our lives (see Appendix A). Yet most staff members knew the difference between commitment and fanaticism, and the ones that didn't soon burned themselves out. We saw ourselves as a third force, a constructive alternative to urban violence or drug-centered lives.

The typical Fort Helper, we think, probably had a lesser degree of self-righteousness and was more other-directed than the usual professional — more intent on building resources. Yet we were an unusual hodgepodge! There was an early staff meeting to which one staff member brought one of her "straight" friends as a visitor. After listening to the discussion for half an hour, he suddenly turned to Lothar, wide-eyed, and said, "I just realized something. These people are *the staff!*"

Two of the people most vital to the success of Fort Help were Helen Garvy and Meg Holmberg. Helen had most recently founded and led an alternative school in San Francisco. Before that she was an organizer and leader of Students for a Democratic Society. Energetic, competent, intelligent, quiet, and strongly independent, she drove herself and sought to inspire others to do everything from sawing and hammering to leading and problem solving. Meg Holmberg, like Helen, in her mid-twenties when the Center for Solving Problems started, graduated in psychology from Swarthmore, and worked as a press aide in both the Eugene McCarthy presidential and the Allard Lowenstein congressional campaigns. She was the "rock" upon which this particular "church" was built, providing our day-to-day coordination, a full-time commitment, and a personal example of altruism and compassion. From the beginnings of our dream in 1969 until June 1975, she counseled, recruited, trained, raised funds, contacted licensing and Medi-Cal agencies, supervised, and conducted the weekly open house with other staff members.

Of the some five hundred people who were part of Fort Help for varying lengths of time and at different levels of contribution over a ten-year period, only a few were actively providing direct help to guests (the term preferred to "clients") during most of this time. As time went by, Joel turned over more leadership functions, including decision making, to other staff. Meg, Lothar, Helen, and a few others were involved in the operation of the center and the helping process itself from the early days. Several of these people continue today as part-time active consultants after years of full-time involvement. Some who had part-time commitments in the earlier years are still functioning as consultants today, also. Only a small number of people have been able, in terms of motivation, financial sacrifice, and stamina, to remain with the center in one capacity or another during its entire history.

INTEGRATING THE EFFORTS

The efforts of this tremendously heterogeneous crew were held together in the early stages by the vision of one man. Had any of us dared step back and take a realistic look at what was going on we would have been bound to say "but this is impossible" and never come back. But Joel is the kind of person who can make one accept innovation and uncertainty as not just inevitable but creative. We believed him when he said that the empty space would shortly be replaced by an attractive "living room," a comprehensive social program, and that we would all soon be doing valuable work. We continued to believe even when the realization of the dream crawled. Part of it was no doubt because few of us had anything to lose, and an incomplete or tardy dream was better than nothing. But most of the success that evolved came out of his perseverance and faith in these ideas and in the abilities of those who had decided to work with him.

THE IDEAS

The primary purpose of Fort Help was and is to provide holistic, humane, and individual help to people with drug, sex, suicide and other special problems (see Appendix B). It began with idealism, commitment, knowledge, and people, rather than money, buildings, equipment, and regulations.

We envisaged Fort Help as a bridge over the increasing fragmentation of American society. Rather than catering to separate groups, such as hippies, blacks, the middle class, or one neighborhood, we hoped to reach out to everyone. Insofar as possible, ours was to be a program analogous in its fields to those of the Mayo and Menninger clinics. Joel stated the dream once in a 1970 newsletter (see Appendix C).

FOUR PREMISES

We started Fort Help with a number of premises. Four were basic. The first was our nonmedical model. We avoided concepts like illness, disturbed, and sick for problems that could be solved. Our model was to emphasize seeking *social* health rather than a simplistic, narrow concept of mental health. We eliminated the pathological frame of reference, with its labeling and stigmatizing. We preferred the term *guest* to *client*. Our staff saw those who came for help as individual human beings, seeking aid in one area of their lives. We envisioned ourselves as an interdisciplinary, eclectic staff of greeters, problem solvers, helpers, and culture workers, rather than psychiatrists, psychologists, or social workers. The medical and psychopathological orientation of mental-health professionals sometimes can lead to the harmful illusion that diagnosis means "I understand you, the patient, and I, the professional, am in control." Our nonmedical model gave Fort Help a different orientation. We felt our time would be better spent trying to understand the unique person and his or her interaction with the major social forces of family, peers, and society. We also rejected the psychopathological orientation because a reasonable fear of being stigmatized keeps many troubled people from seeking help. We realize that many people need to believe in a dogmatic psychological, religious, or political philosophy, and that some people feel comfortable only with traditional formalities and medical paraphenalia. Nevertheless, we were to work for people not institutions, and we favored individual self-determination over adjustment to the status quo. Fort Help was intended to be a different model of health care: human, accessible, open to all regardless of ability to pay, comprehensive, oriented toward keeping people well, and making maximum use of paraprofessionals.

Our second basic premise, which follows from the above, is that one does not necessarily have to be a mental health professional in order to help people.

Anyone with relevant life experience, maturity, skills, and commitment could join our staff, on which there was to be no differentiation based on titles, degrees, age, sex, or race. We forged a new organizational style, in a voluntary association of people dedicated to solving problems in a nonhierarchical, nonauthoritarian, status-free manner. We saw ourselves doing what needs to be done, privately and without profit, without bureaucratic buck-passing, inefficiency, and dehumanization.

Thus the third premise, intricately connected with the other two in our planning of the center, is that there should be no hierarchy, no differentiation based on diverse skills. Rather, we wanted a participatory democracy in which not only everyone contributed, but one in which it was possible to develop and maintain a standard of excellence at the same time.

Our plan for a participatory democracy was intimately linked to our fourth premise, what we called "the smorgasbord approach." This approach was intended to make Fort Help an eclectic and innovative helping facility — blending every traditional and new technique from psychotherapy and encounter groups to hypnosis, massage, and music. Long before the concept of holistic gained currency, Fort Help aimed to help the total person through a wide range of methods: evaluation, detoxification, methadone and antabuse, medication for heroin addicts and alcoholics, casework, brief therapy and crisis intervention, social-work services, vocational counseling, medico-legal evaluation and court testimony, individual counseling and therapy, family therapy, group therapy, psychodrama and role playing, sensitivity and encounter groups, behavior therapy, hypnosis, music and art therapy, self-help including the use of Alcoholics Anonymous and Daytop-Synanon techniques, community outreach including satellite help centers, and home visits.

Throughout the history of Fort Help, one of the most strongly observed rules has been the total absence of an official method of helping. Some staff members would have preferred a single focus, such as psychotherapy. In our "sociatric" rather than psychiatric approach, we presented this smorgasbord of help. We often allowed the person being helped to choose among our techniques; we usually combined two or more methods for each guest.

THE ENVIRONMENT

Fort Help was and is an implicit model for renewing the past and creating the future. In addition to larger concerns, we gave much thought to our physical environment: 1) a central location in San Francisco and the Bay Area not identified with any one minority or majority group; 2) rented space to avoid large capital expenditures and the time-consuming, sometimes degrading, seeking of large funds; 3) low rent; 4) easy access by car, public transportation, and telephone (by arranging for easily remembered numbers, such as 864-HELP and, later, UNI-SEX-5); 5) brightly colored and curved walls, simple and modern furniture, plants, and paintings to create an informal, warm atmosphere; 6) no distracting phones in counseling (helping) rooms; 7) no rooms for administration and personal offices (overhead was decreased; all space was available for direct help; moreover, any status defined by who had which office was eliminated); 8) both freshly prepared and vending-machine refreshments; 9) flexible hours (including nights, weekends, and holidays); 10) flexible, affordable fees, which were discussed only after immediate help was provided at the first visit; 11) convenient scheduling of appointments, including drop-ins; 12) no forms to fill out or requirements to be met; 13) no records required, or even a name, if the person preferred anonymity or a pseudonym.

In summary, we envisaged democratic decision making, equality, tolerance, eclecticism and flexibility. We sought to avoid the negative features characteristic of many traditional bureaucratic organizations. Moreover, we wanted to overcome the barriers that frequently develop between counselor and "patient," between those who can pay and those who cannot, between administrators and staff, between city and suburbs. We were one staff, finding fulfillment without titles, without personal offices, and without much money.

CHAPTER 2

BUILDING THE DREAM: REALITY

The shortest and surest way to live with honor . . . is to be in reality what we would appear to be. —Socrates

As a specific entity, the National Center for Solving Special Social and Health Problems, or FORT HELP (nonmilitary, perhaps the only such "fort" in the U.S.), began in late 1969. As noted earlier, Joel first thought of some of its important concepts and built them into a government program, the San Francisco Department of Health's Center for Special Problems, in 1965. However, the testing and proving of the premises, their unforeseen ramifications and the surprising opposition from the general social welfare community, comprised much of the experience and organizational history of Fort Help.

DEVELOPING THE FACILITY

Since the building on Howard Street had no interior walls, we put much effort into construction. An imaginative architect with a talent for interesting unconventional design, Seth Curlin, experimented with the available forty-six hundred square feet of free-flowing space. The staff did the actual carpentry work ourselves. We built most of the walls so that they would be curved and meet at odd angles. We accomplished this time-consuming task, prohibitively expensive at the prevailing pay scales for union labor, even though we were unskilled at carpentry, construction, plumbing, or wiring. We learned how to bend, flange, and cantilever. We also learned that there are certain things that *cannot* be done by people who barely know one end of a hammer from the other. Many design ideas were compromised — for one, after many months of slow progress, a number of rooms were quickly built with straight walls simply because they were urgently needed. But the overall architecture was original and attractive enough to give us a feeling this was indeed a special place. Our place on Howard Street was a marked contrast to what we felt were drab and Kafkaesque hospitals, government buildings, and "free" clinics known to most seekers of help.

Our 1970 newsletter on "Creating the Space" told of the successful efforts to get a city building permit, rehabilitate the electrical and plumbing services, put on a new roof, and clean up the place. Some of the space remained open for a time, to allow us to experiment with different movable partitions, interview groupings, and treatment situations. Everyone involved with Fort Help actively shaped it by contributing hundreds of hours of work. Everyone helped to stretch our budget: pay less for an item, donate an item, or help to pay for one personally. We needed typewriters, folding tables, duplicating machine and supplies, a truck or van for a future mobile unit, chairs, lamps, carpets, door frames and doors, lighting and plumbing fixtures, and paint (eventually donated by the Zelinsky Paint Company).

Money was a problem. Joel contributed a sizable amount of his own limited "public practice" income to the center during the early months, in addition to his time, to build what we had planned and to help pay for other essential expenses such as telephones and utilities. Even with volunteer labor, it did take about twenty thousand dollars to achieve our environmental ideals.

But the place functioned well, most of the time. There was something exciting about making do with very little, bringing concepts to life, and proving that money and bigness weren't everything.

FORMAL STRUCTURES

Even an antibureaucratic, futuristic program such as Fort Help must become involved with government to the extent of obtaining the necessary permits. Although these were minimal and usually not of our choice, each was time-consuming. Sometimes getting the required license was a demoralizing experience, incompatible with our ethical philosophy. The 1972 Medi-Cal connection with the California State Department of Public Health, and its aftermath, almost destroyed us as an organization. First came the formalities of incorporation as a nonprofit, tax-exempt organization. Although we started the procedures early, it wasn't until October 1971 that the I. R. S. formalized our status. Next came the relatively simple inspection and approval by the state health department that formalized us as a community clinic.

In order to receive federal and state approval as a nonprofit group, the center needed a board of directors. In addition to Joel, our directors included Willie Brown, California assemblyman and majority leader (at the time of this writing); Owen Chamberlain, Nobel Prize-winning professor of physics at the University of California, Berkeley; Howard Craven, Bank of America vice-president; June Oppen Degnan, treasurer of the Eugene McCarthy campaign for president; Victor di Suvero, businessman and writer; Alvin Duskin, environmentalist; the Reverend Ted McIlvenna; Jerry Mander, advertising executive; Stephanie Mills, birth control activist; Richard Moore, president of the local public television station KQED and filmmaker; Arthur Morgan, U.S. Department of Agriculture scientist; Charles O'Brien, former California chief deputy attorney general; Dorothy Patterson, nurse; and the Reverend Cecil Williams, pastor of Glide Memorial Church. Later the board also included Don Chamberlin, radio talk show host; John F. Connelly, Jr.; Maria Fort, Office of Economic Opportunity official; Richard Hongisto, sheriff (at the time) of San Francisco; Robert Kantor, attorney; Art Lantz, attorney; Toni Rembe, attorney; Arthur Rock, investor; Lothar Salin, staff; Karen Stone, principal of the private Nueva Day School; William Soskin, psychologist; and Cecil Whitebone, San Francisco automobile dealer.

OPENING

The early idyll was not to last. People were rapidly hearing about us, starting to call us, and even dropping by in significant numbers. There was no formal opening or press conference. As people asked for help, we provided it to whomever might come in, even though we weren't ready with all the comprehensive services we had planned. Eventually, we set an arbitrary date of November 6, 1970, for the official announcement of what we had already been doing. A San Francisco *Chronicle* reporter visited us and wrote a story ("Unorthodox S.F. Center, A Nice Place to Get Help," *San Francisco Chronicle*, Tuesday, November 10, 1970) which had the effect of flooding us with people who needed help for their personal problems. Fully ready or not, we were open.

EARLY BEGINNINGS

Originally there was no electricity; our night staff-meetings were held in eerie candlelight, as were some of our early night sessions with guests. Neither was there a central heating system. During the first winter we had a large and somewhat noisy gas-fueled contraption that generated a wall of hot air in the main lobby. Later on, we brought a few small electric room heaters. A heating system was not installed until the end of our second winter. The first two years at Fort Help proved that much can be done in spite of limited resources. Our toilet facilities were integrated and workable.

In addition to the main lobby, there were then a total of six counseling rooms, ranging from small cubicles to those accommodating a sizable group. We also had a holding area, good for brief conferences, behind a large, curved room divider. A back room became usable when stored building material was pushed aside. Of these nine areas, at least two usually would be unavailable at any one time, for one reason or another. Since we did not use a room reservation system then and did not have enough rooms, there was always a scramble among us for the rooms that were available. In spite of this, most counseling sessions were held as scheduled, even if it sometimes meant that different groups would be crowded together or a single guest would be seen in a cavernous group room. On occasion we even held sessions in our cars.

At the front of the main lobby, we made certain that someone was present at the receiving desk, where the duties ranged from merely giving general directions and answering phones to doing the equivalent of intake and referral work. It was one of the most tedious jobs at the center.

The original "vault" had become a staff room. The two long walls had been faced with shallow plywood tables, covered with telephones and telephone books, files, forms, and notes. Giving immediate help by telephone was a top priority. We sat at the table in safari chairs, some of us giving telephone help-advice in brief, half-hour installments, some of us making appointments, and some taking care of personal calls, since this small area was the only place to catch our breath between guests or to exchange professional confidentialities. The traffic was always thick. The solid concrete walls created an occasionally unpleasant acoustic reverberation.

Our plan for the first stage of operation was basically simple. Rather than have an understaffed facility with extended hours, we condensed the operation into three afternoons and evenings during the week. We gave additional help over the telephone, hoping to supplement this help later by a mobile van. On Mondays, Wednesdays, and Saturdays we opened our doors from noon to at least 8 P.M., followed by a staff meeting. On Saturday mornings, we conducted staff training. Until the center was fully operational, the service slots on these three days were taken by groups of people who wanted to work together, who knew and trusted each other. This was our concept of *primary groups*.

Each working day had its own primary group. Some members, endowed with a great deal of energy and time, belonged to two or even three primary groups; they were at the center several times a week. Before too long, the groups were meeting on Tuesdays and Thursdays, although nothing was initially planned for those days and evenings. In the beginning, "everyone" was accepted as part of the staff; anyone who showed up regularly and participated in the group development sessions could help at the Fort. Later each person shared responsibility for colleague selection, on-the-job training and supervision, and general problem solving.

Under our concept of participatory democracy, no one was to make arbitrary decisions involving work to be done without accepting the responsibility of actually *doing* it (not necessarily alone). All of us had dealt with too many administrators whose days revolve around thinking only of things for *others* to do! It worked exceedingly well during the summer of 1970, since there were no deadlines. There were *shared* tasks in construction, fund raising, staff training, telephone services, and support work that went on without a sophisticated PERT flowchart. There was always something to do and people interested in doing it with enthusiasm.

Along with eliminating the need for administrators, we eliminated the need for secretaries and clerks. This action seemed to increase service time while simultaneously dramatically decreasing paperwork. When people equally share in typing memos and letters, phone work, sorting mail, errands, and cleaning up, there is both less bureaucracy and better morale.

A semi-monthly general meeting of all staff helpers gave the first overall direction to the center's operation. An agenda for this meeting was prepared in advance to assure coverage of important items; but adequate time for nonagenda items was made available. At the general meeting three coordinators were selected to supervise, in consultation with Joel, the day-to-day operation of the center. They served staggered, renewable terms of two and three months. All three had to have been fully cleared by the other staff members for unsupervised counseling. The coordinators identified a number of necessary administrative functions and submitted to the general meeting for its review the names of "activators" to carry out these functions. This was to be an *ad hoc* structure which was expected to shift with changing needs. Coordinators and activators prepared the agenda for the general meeting, to which each reported at least once a month.

Once we began full operations, our organizing capability was drastically reduced. Providing direct help was our first priority. Time had to be kept available for guests during the times when the center was open. Furthermore, since many of the staff members needed outside activities to make a living, they could not be expected to give up an additional evening every week to participate in organizational decisions.

The inherent weaknesses of centralized authority are lack of communication and involvement. On the other hand, a fully participatory process can break down under the sheer weight of time required to reach agreement on even the most trivial matters. A rational system must avoid both extremes. However, no system will work except in an atmosphere of trust and respect. At Fort Help we jettisoned the bureaucracy while trying to maintain a rational system.

For the first six months, we absorbed almost one hundred percent of everybody's efforts and energy in building services, leadership, and facilities simultaneously. We had arrived at the spring of 1970. Months of ideas and planning had gone by. The flower children had come to San Francisco's Haight-Ashbury in the late Sixties, and they had wilted — their petals plucked by dope dealers and reporters. The needs of thousands of thoroughly alienated young people with manifold drug and sometimes criminal problems, along with the continuing needs of the poor and middle class, swamped the traditional public health services and private practices of the community. Some of their needs remained neglected. In our search for new and better ways to meet those needs, we began the long, bureaucratic process of obtaining the "wonder drug," methadone, for the growing numbers of narcotic addicts. Methadone was intended to free people from physical dependency on heroin while they received counseling for their social and emotional problems. We wanted our methadone program to be part of a full range of services for sexual, drug, suicide, criminal, and other human problems. Everyone — addict and nonaddict, homosexual and heterosexual, hip and straight — would be offered hope and treatments.

DIVISION OF LABOR

We felt it to be essential that helping services be performed only by individuals qualified in the following categories:

1. Generalist: able to work independently, with a variety of problems, on a one-to-one counseling or group leadership basis, on a long- or short-term basis.

2. Specialist: skilled in a specific field in which one is able to work unsupervised (may also be apprenticed in other categories).

3. Indirect helper: works in office, construction, newsletter, fund raising, and similar services.

4. Trainee: training in chosen fields under specific supervisors; may work at selected tasks under supervision.

To avoid the medically oriented, bureaucratic jargon of the mental health field, and what we felt to be the harmful effects of thus labeling people, we introduced the terms *greeter*, *problem solver*, and *guest*. Only the first of these remained in use and became an accepted, everyday term, although *helper* has had intermittent use. *Problem solver* was never popular and was soon replaced by *generalist*, which eventually yielded to *counselor*. Everyone agreed that *patient* was bad, but *guest* proved uncomfortable for many; therefore, *client* was most often substituted as a half-way term, even though Joel derided the term. Most of all we stressed that it was not necessary to call those who came for help by anything but their chosen personal name. We even gave the rooms individual names with positive concepts (Joy, Peace, Happiness, Relief) to escape the anonymity and sterility of numbered cubicles.

Another key part of the "open staff" idea was its two categories: *direct* services (helping and other contacts with guests) and *indirect* services (everything else). Anyone performing indirect services could get further training and become apprenticed to a counselor so that he or she could become a helper, too. Since neither category could function without the other, both were equally valuable. Every staff member had an opportunity to excel at *something* (and often several things).

Since we never seemed to have enough experienced generalists, the greeter-/problem solver was designated the first line of service staff and the generalist-/counselor the backup, in a modification of the original plan. Many of the greeters were *experienced* and highly capable, but *lacked depth and training* when they came to see us; it was essentially left to them to decide which people and problems were to be cared for on the spot and which were to be referred for more in-depth work. However, such responsibility soon led to problems in defining the greeter's task. Thus a 1971 newsletter reports on a "greeter workshop" held a few days previously:

> The Greeter-Problem Solver was originally intended to be more than a welcoming committee or someone to make appointments from the desk. In truth persons coming to us for help were never supposed to be received by someone behind a *desk*. The Greeter was seen as someone with sufficient training and experience to be able to recognize the problems of the client and what services available at Fort Help or elsewhere would most fulfill his needs. The greeter was also conceived as one capable of doing short term, basic problem-solving counseling. And underlying all this is the idea that any person coming to Fort Help could get *immediate* competent help with his problem without getting involved in a bureaucratic tangle. These goals have not always been realized in the past (year). This has been partly due to the fact that new Greeters are often people with high potential but little counseling experience who never received the proper orientation or training to be able to function effectively. There has also been a failure to properly define the roles of various new staff members with regard to making the distinction between greeters and staff serving in indirect services.

Not surprisingly, then, there were some generalists who considered greeters to be little more than intake clerks, while some of the greeters felt they could handle more problems than were assigned to them. Eventually, the greeters gained both more experience and the upper hand in decision-making proceedings, and incorporated the generalist concept into their helping approach.

In organizing tasks to be done by many people, it is traditional to have job descriptions and assignments. We attempted to do without these establishment trappings by emphasizing cooperation, voluntary choice, and peer-group evaluation and support. Most of the time and in most respects this worked well. It certainly provided a more creative, spontaneous work atmosphere. Nevertheless, major problems arose in two obvious areas:

1. The basic premise for our large staff and its many tasks was that people would choose those ones that they would like to do, resulting in everything getting done without anyone having to do something he or she didn't like. However, it turns out that there are always some things no one wants to do. Also, sometimes, someone tires of a task he or she has been doing, and wishes someone else would take it over.

2. We *assumed* that the tasks people chose to do also were ones they were capable of doing, and that their own good sense of responsibility as well as potential peer-group disapproval would control this. Sometimes our assumptions were wrong and these control mechanisms failed to work.

ATTRACTING AND ASSESSING STAFF

A process of peer-group assessment was our way of staff selection and assignment, our more open and democratic equivalent of the screening of personnel elsewhere. It was a simple idea. Groups of twelve or fifteen members met together and decided among themselves just what each of them would be doing at the center, based on both past experience and what they had observed about each other's abilities. This implied a limitation on what some people could do, but a few thought this was too "authoritarian." So, it was up to each person to tell the group what services he or she felt capable of performing, and why. The group then decided in his or her presence, with an opportunity for discussion, what they felt to be acceptable tasks for that person. Each person's mutually agreed-upon services and restrictions were then listed on a file card, for reference when needed.

When the initial group of staff members had gone through the assessment process and been assigned suitable duties and limitations, we established a regular process for screening and accepting new staff members. Our regular newsletter outlined this process:

"PLUGGING IN" TO FORT HELP

As the word spreads and interest in the Center increases, more and more new people are coming to the staff meetings. It's good to have new faces and fresh enthusiasm, but when the Center is open, this may be somewhat disruptive. To be sure that new people get a chance to find out about the Center in a relaxed informal setting, we'd like to encourage first-time visitors to Fort Help to drop in between 6 and 8 p.m. on Mondays for Open House. At that time, staff members will be available to tell people about the Center, answer questions, and talk with prospective volunteers (and those seeking help) about the Center's operations and philosophy. By having all new volunteers come at this time each week, we can keep the staff free at other times to concentrate on their helping and training activities.

Following the Open House, anyone interested in working at the Center should fill out an Interest & Skills Survey form and talk with the Training Coordinator about getting into a training session. If, after attending several training sessions and getting to know the Center staff, a person feels he/she would like to commit to working at the Center, a group of staff members will meet with her or him to assess their experience and skills and determine specific responsibilities.

Hopefully this procedure will provide a smooth means of absorbing new staff into the Center's activities and putting their skills and interest to work as quickly as possible.

The drop-in open house and the open organization concepts have continued to the present time. The only additional change in this procedure was that before long a special committee (work group) was established to deal with assessment on an ongoing basis. It has been a part of the Fort Help operation ever since. While there were general criteria for assessment, the assessment committee had almost total leeway in interpreting them. Unfortunately, like the conventional civil service/personnel systems, these criteria could be used to screen out anyone who did not fit the biases of the particular committee members at any one time. However, people were encouraged to directly discuss the assessment decisions with the group, who had to give detailed reasons for their decisions. Moreover, rejected applicants could appeal a rejection to the overall staff. They could also reapply in three months.

The questionnaire that was used to guide the committee in making preliminary decisions covered such items as the applicant's experience and training; what he or she wanted out of his or her experience at Fort Help, and what he or she was planning to contribute. Originally, we planned to interview everyone who submitted an application, since we considered it bureaucratic and inadequate to judge anyone on the basis of a questionnaire alone. In practice, however, we soon found a close relationship between a paper impression and a personal evaluation. We eventually found ourselves with a four-month backlog of applications, which probably led to our losing a number of talented potential staff members. The decision was made to interview in person only those applicants whose written documentation appealed to the majority of the assessment committee members (at least three of the five). This plan, too, has remained in effect ever since.

Peer group assessment, therefore, designated some staff members for certain kinds of services and barred others from doing things for which they were not qualified. Once this procedure was established, we added new people after fairly rigorous screening by the democratically selected assessment committee.

New staff members were assigned to the same work categories and limitations as their seniors. The rule was that, before starting to work at something for which one was not assessed, the committee had to be informed and give its approval to the change. A portion of the staff called this set-up "bureaucratic" or even "fascist," claiming that, left to themselves, everyone would act responsibly and not exceed their capacities. While this sounded good, we found that in practice it did not necessarily follow.

In fact, by the spring of 1971, we became aware that some staff members were ignoring their assessment limitations. Those who were assigned to perform indirect services only were counseling the guests; those who were cleared to be group co-leaders were doing one-to-one counseling; and some who should have been giving advice on how to stop smoking were involved in such therapy as psychodrama. There was even one person who came in every Wednesday night to lead a group without ever having been assessed. (Everyone presumed he had been cleared to be a member of the staff — our first and only impersonator!) Although the overwhelming majority of staff performed competently and responsibly, there were enough members performing non-approved tasks that corrective action had to be taken.

We decided that the entire group, including Joel, would go through a reassessment process of interview and review by three other staff members. Those who had been found to have exceeded their original assignments but were found also to be capable of what they were now doing were cleared. If found not capable, they would have to limit themselves to their assignments. With a staff of almost one hundred, this was a time-consuming process but it took place largely in an atmosphere of good will. Once more this showed a creative, if revolutionary, path. (Can you imagine what would happen in the traditional bureaucracy if everybody had to undergo a regular reassessment and peer review in order to keep their jobs?) However, some of those who were found to have significantly exceeded their limitations tried to circumvent the inevitable. They agitated for the establishment of a totally open staff where everyone, staff and guest alike, would be allowed to do whatever he or she felt qualified for, limited only by the right of others to confront them on what they were doing. To our credit, they were not supported.

In May 1971, the assessment group presented its reassessment plan to the staff via the newsletter. In addition to the reassessment process, the group would determine which staff members were active; find consultants within the staff for other staff members who needed more training; and, in general, spot any problems that might exist within the current staff.

These were the ground rules for reassessment, as outlined by the assessment committee: 1) Each of the members of the assessment committee will take responsibility for interviewing some of the staff, with staff members having the option of meeting with the entire assessment committee. 2) The basic questions to be asked are listed, but the interviews will not be limited to just those questions. It was suggested that every staff member prepare answers to the questions before the actual interview. 3) At the end of each interview, the interviewer's feelings and conclusions will be communicated directly to the interviewed staff member(s) before any statement is taken back to the assessment committee. These were our questions:

1. What will be your time commitment to Fort Help in the next three months; the next six months?

2. What are your present responsibilities at Fort Help? How do these relate to what you were assessed to do?

3. Are you providing consultation for anyone on the staff? Are you receiving consultation?

4. What do you do well; what do you have problems doing?

5. List problem areas (suicide, sex, drugs including alcohol and tobacco, etc.) that you are interested in working in and those in which you need training.

6. Which techniques are you skilled in; which would you like to learn?

7. In view of your personal vision of what Fort Help should be, what would you do as a leader to bring that vision about? What do you think are the ideal qualities and actions of the decision makers, leaders, or leadership?

8. Open question: Do you have any other comments or suggestions on any subject not covered here?

The guidelines were followed, but the process required months rather than the hoped-for weeks.

DEMOCRATIC LEADERSHIP AND HELP ("THERAPY")

Although Joel had not envisioned the center as a place where separate administrators made all the decisions and the front-line workers were treated as peons, Fort Help was not planned to be an anarchy or a "workers' collective." We came to realize that a place cannot run itself without admitting to and sharing certain minimal administrative work.

In the earliest days, when helping services were being phased in gradually, many of the *de facto* leaders of the center were either untrained counselor-therapists or people who had little initial interest in doing administrative work. The staff as a whole remained in ultimate control, but the coordinators handled day-to-day operations. As noted earlier, functional limitations for all staff members were set and defined, with a right of appeal for those who felt they had cause for complaint, and most importantly, the assessment process and quality control of services were placed firmly in the hands of a committee made up of a majority of generalists. This organizational model reached an almost optimal compromise between intra-staff openness and democracy on the one hand and quality of services on the other. Unfortunately, given the openness and freedom at Fort Help, agreeing on something was not the same as making sure it was always followed.

RESPONSIBILITY

Fifteen significant task areas were outlined, of which six were assigned to Joel and nine had no specific person-in-charge. There is an inevitable conflict between standards of output and the amount of democratic freedom in operation. If no one is accountable to anyone but himself or herself and his or her peers, some people will do outstanding work but others will do little. Meg Holmberg, at that point in her life, was largely interested in community organizing, as was C., a talented, very competent, single parent and former "radical." R., T., and L. were interested in fund raising and public education; J., a degreed social worker, wanted to organize the planned mobile-help unit similar to the one Joel and she had developed and operated in the city's anti-poverty program. These women, along with Joel, were the main powers in the loosely organized coordinating committee that met weekly to decide what happened next.

Members of the direct service-oriented staff were also part of the coordinating group, which was open to all staff members, but their attendance at meetings was sporadic and hence their leadership voice less significant. There was A., the head of the Haight-Ashbury Switchboard, who coined the name "FORT HELP"; R., a Ph.D. candidate in psychology who showed administrative skill as well as energy; and F., whose principal interest was in helping to establish the planned sex clinic. Others who participated in the coordinating decisions were M., an experienced therapist and leader in the homosexual community, whom Joel had previously brought into the Center for Special Problems; J., a promising graduate student at San Francisco State University; J., a sociologist and Navy veteran; and Lothar, both an experienced manager and group facilitator. There was deliberately no authoritarian, pyramidal, hierarchical organization chart — the group was expected to function on a team basis. Most of the time this went on smoothly and with much more enthusiasm than at meetings in later years.

EARLY PROGRESS REPORT

The original document on Joel's vision (Appendix C), setting forth the scope of the proposed center, reveals a common theme among the problems to be solved: the problems are pervasive, societal in origin with only secondary psychological features, and require new approaches since the old ones have failed. At a coordinators' meeting in September, 1971, Joel presented a detailed paper in which he summed up his impatience about some things that were going on. He started by restating what the center should be doing and continued with a list of accomplishments and problems (Appendix C), adding the comment "I think our accomplishments are at least equal to our problems in importance."

His principal impatience was with the fact that many of the things he had wanted to see at the center were still not reality: no relationship counseling, no alcoholism program, nothing to help people stop smoking — in addition to which a few staff themselves smoked in violation of our basic policy. Actually some relationship counseling was being conducted and would be sharply expanded later on, and alcoholism work was done sporadically when we had someone on the staff to do it. Anti-smoking programs were created later, when Joel started putting some personal energy into doing them and into training the few other interested staff members. Sleeplessness, gambling, and death-and-dying programs never went beyond the stages of minimal staff training, special seminars, and discussion, and of counseling a small number of individuals with these problems.

CORE GROUP

As we continued to try different forms of democracy, leadership at the Fort gradually evolved into what we called a "core group." We began to have regular weekly staff meetings to handle new or difficult matters. Decisions were generally made by a majority of the ten or twelve members (the core of a staff of fifty) who came to a particular meeting. We used an informal process of self-selection for this core group, thereby reducing the loss of staff time and energy put into the many general staff meetings before. In the beginning, the core group met away from the center in order to have freedom of discussion without interruption by the operations.

Almost casually, this core group came up with what turned out to be a drastic policy change. It decided that since there was so much more work to be done with the steadily increasing numbers of people seeking help, only those who could spend at least ten hours weekly would be considered staff members. Everyone else, no matter how long they had been at Fort Help, would either be asked to leave or would become a non-voting consultant, respected but excluded from the decision-making process. Like many changes in organizations or societies, the full implications of it had not been envisaged. Those who were excluded from the staff turned out to be some of the most skilled — people who had been donating half a dozen hours or an evening out of a busy schedule, a full-time job, or a private practice. Their departure lowered the level of staff competence and, with it, the overall quality of the work for a time.

In addition, the core group made a major revision of staff functions. In the beginning, it will be recalled, our idea had been that people with different talents would all contribute what they could, and that one kind of work would be considered as valuable as another. In addition, some people were permitted to work independently, while others could do so only as apprentices under supervision. Some people concentrated on longer-term help of guests with drug, sex, suicide, or other major problems; some were specialists in greeting and health-oriented, short-term crisis counseling; some had mainly administrative duties. Now everyone was supposed to do some of the same kind of work as everyone else. The new policy gradually took hold, though not without long, bitter fights. From the summer of 1973 to the fall of 1974, core group meetings were largely struggles over the proper orientation for the staff. Heavy emphasis was now placed on telephone crisis work. At this time, less than a majority of staff were capable of intensive work with guests.

One of the corollaries of this change in policy was that staff members were held more accountable for doing a minimum amount of work. Everyone was required to spend a certain number of hours at the center. In order to get the minimal stipend ($50 weekly), one had to be there twenty hours weekly, spending time productively, and monitoring his or her own responsibility. However, overall checks were made on how much time everyone spent on telephone help. Now the staff decided that in order to get a stipend one had to meet minimal standards of productive work and fees for counseling sessions. A survey showed that some people were being paid without seeing a single guest, and others were not collecting any fees for their services. As a result, several people lost their stipends.

There was also a change of process. When it was discovered that some people who had been accepted on the staff were performing without supervision, groups were started to make sure that everyone was at least receiving peer consultation and review. After a while, participation in such a group was made mandatory. In April 1975, a consultant group was established to review staff abilities and to advise the staff meetings on quality of care.

As a result, Fort Help became increasingly work-oriented and more careful (sometimes too careful) about admitting new people to staff. There was also a change in criteria for accepting new people for the staff. Without any fanfare, the concept of *apprenticeship*, which had been with us from the start, was dropped. People were accepted who were felt to be fully qualified to work without supervision. One was either on staff or not and, if so, was encouraged to try new things and to be responsible.

With surprisingly little resistance the staff accepted these recommendations as policy. They realized that there were some very talented people from whom one could learn something and that a reasonable amount of supervision was desirable.

It speaks for the vitality of Fort Help and for the sturdiness of its founding concepts that the center evolved to become both better and smaller. Lothar had been one of the first among the staff to seek an "academic seal of approval" for his ability and experience. Now a growing proportion of others found their way not only into informal programs such as Goddard's but also into more structured ones at Lone Mountain College, the California School of Professional Psychology, the state universities, and even the School of Social Work at the University of California, Berkeley. Students also started to use the center as a field placement for doctoral and masters studies, as well as for internships and residencies.

Chapter 3
FURTHER GLIMPSES INTO
PROGRAMS AND OPERATIONS

There's nothing more difficult to carry out, more doubtful of success, more dangerous, than to initiate a new order of things. For the reformer has enemies in all those who profit by the old order, and only lukewarm defenders in all those who profit by the new. —Machiavelli

Because there were so many components to our dream, the inevitable compromises kept parts of it from becoming a reality. Financial shortage was a constant problem because we offered no commercially attractive treatments which would induce people to "buy"; neither did we create artificial charismatic media figures to attract fame or wealth. After moderate to lengthy periods of service, most people left the staff because we stressed that they should not define their worth through lifelong participation in one organization, and because they could not be expected to make indefinite financial and status sacrifices. Self interest on the parts of some of our own staff members, general societal apathy and ingratitude, and a few establishment bureaucrats from other agencies made a small number of our goals impossible to fulfill. Most of our goals were attained, however, and can be extrapolated not only to other government and private organizations but to the broader society as well.

PROGRAMS

Antiaddiction and Methadone Maintenance Program

The guest population for methadone services varied from a high of 130 to a low of 70. Depending to some extent on changing government regulations and on their own progress, most of these people at first came in for their dosage every day or every other day, and all at least twice a week. The staff consisted of one or two full-time nurses doing the first-line contact and dispensing; a part-time physician supervising dosage and performing those other legally required functions for which a medical license is needed; and three or four half-time staff members, including ex-addicts of both sexes, who covered a range of duties from counseling to record keeping and taking the urine samples required by the government.

The cost of this methadone program has been consistently less than $100,000 per year, with an average of $7,000-$8,000 monthly. Fort Help is a model of what can be accomplished with methadone realistically at a respectable cost-efficiency ratio. Government methadone programs seem to result in large numbers of doctors, nurses, counselors, and secretaries, with large salaries and fringe benefits, who must be supervised by many administrators. The Fort Help methadone program, as much as any part of our operation, proved that an innovative organization without administrators and government interference can provide services effectively, with dignity to the recipients, and at a reasonable cost. It is a matter of some pride that a State of California review team, which assessed our operation carefully during the summer of 1976, came to essentially the same conclusion, saying, in effect, "we don't know how you're doing it but you're doing a damned good job."

In the 1950s methadone was used to treat the withdrawal illness of heroin addiction, and in general medicine, as an analgesic alternative to morphine and Demerol. It is easy to establish and maintain in a steady dosage because it is long acting (more than twelve hours per dose), it can be taken orally rather than intravenously without losing any effectiveness, and it will block the effects of heroin. This means that someone on a steady maintenance regimen of methadone will experience little or no benefit from heroin and have no reason to seek it. An addict can get methadone from legal programs, at low cost, in pure form, and have to take it only once a day, rather than injecting highly impure street heroin several times a day at a cost of $100-$200 daily.

However, there are important philosophical and ethical questions involved in deciding to use such a drug at all: Given the facts that our multibillion dollar federal, state, and city agencies have failed miserably to stop the flow of narcotics and other drugs into this country, that these drugs are expensive to obtain, and that addicts engage in numerous burglaries and assaults to obtain money for heroin, then the legal dispensing of methadone appears to have a sound rationale. Heroin, contrary to popular belief, has no lasting physical effects on the user and should itself also be available legally for limited maintenance use. But heroin was long ago (1920s) needlessly barred from American physicians by the Federal Bureau of Narcotics.

Our basic rationale, then, for the legal dispensing of methadone was as follows: 1) putting an addict on methadone will free him or her from the necessity of engaging in self-destructive and antisocial activities such as prostitution or burglary; 2) in such a situation, the addict will be able to get a job and function socially; and 3) with suitable counseling accompanying the drug maintenance, every addict can in time get to the point of being completely drug-free. In fact, we focused our treatment on the goal of getting off methadone as soon as possible (and staying off heroin), ideally in a maximum of two years.

How effective were we? Of the three goals mentioned above, the first has been considerably successful, the second has been generally successful, and the third has been sometimes successful. The number of addicts who became and also stayed drug-free, including methadone, is small for almost any program nationwide. However, keeping thousands of addicts from self- and social destruction is of great social value. "Success" and "failure" are hard to define and establish, especially on an absolute scale. It may be impossible to achieve total rehabilitation when the unemployment rate is so high in general (more so for ex-addicts and minorities), and when addicts are so stigmatized. Also, whether methadone or alcohol, it is hard for a user to give up a simple chemical remedy for a more complex, long-range solution to problems.

What, then, of methadone maintenance in comparison to other treatment approaches? The principal drawback of the nonresidential Alcoholics Anonymous and the far more authoritarian residential Synanon/Delancey nondrug models, as we see them, is that they create their own societies in which dependency on drugs has been traded for lifelong dependency on the authoritarian (in the case of the live-in groups) support group. Synanon may be successful in eliminating the symptom—drug abuse—but still be a failure in establishing an authentic, independent, socially functioning individual. Methadone, on the other hand, preserves the symptom (albeit legally and more healthily), but enables many people to function normally in society.

Since we are private and not funded by government, the program at Fort Help is able to maintain total anonymity for our guests. We have been able to attract a considerable number of people who, though addicted, are able to go to school, work, and have families. Addicted people *can*, if they are not criminalized by society, lead socially productive, normal lives. Without the legal drug methadone, these same individuals would at the very least be depriving their families of necessities in order to buy heroin, and at worst be stealing, prostituting themselves, or mugging others, or be imprisoned or dead. Providing this service and these benefits consistently for some one hundred motivated people appears to outweigh the disadvantages of also having to work with many addicts who remain poorly adjusted socially, who continue to use some illegal drugs or much alcohol, or whose behavior is a source of irritation.

At one time, most members of our methadone staff were black or chicano. The presence of large numbers of minority people, both as guests and staff, differentiated the methadone program from the rest of Fort Help. Just why the center in its other programs was unable to attract more than small numbers of blacks, Latinos, Asians, and other minorities is not known. The several months of unpaid work required of the staff in the beginning, and the low salaries later, may have discouraged some. Since qualified minority people have good opportunities in mental health clinics and in private practice, they were less likely to work at a place like Fort Help, even though we actively tried to recruit them. On the other hand, Fort Help has been phenomenally successful in breaking all existing barriers of sexism, ageism, and false professionalism.

After much soul-searching, and with great regret, we fired two of our ex-addict male staff members. One of them, a basically violent street person, was doing an admirable job of controlling his anger until he was involved in a fight over a woman. The other man was involved in situations in which money disappeared and, also, in a questionable financial transaction with a guest. While they were with us, though, it meant a great deal to both of them that they had "made it" for at least an extended period of time. Like some of the other Fort Help staff, the ex-addicts proved that one could move from guest to staff member/helper, even if only temporarily.

Most of the time the needs of those guests receiving methadone—dispensing, counseling, medical complaints, job help, making appointments—were taken care of by an increasingly (over the years) separately working methadone staff. When more help was required, particularly for the legally mandated supervision of the weekly urine specimen, the other staff members often gave their time grudgingly. The laboratory testing bill for these analyses is the single largest expense connected with the program and figured prominently in our financial crisis of late 1971. We called this "Operation Golden Flow," derogatorily, and attacked it as unnecessary, expensive, and demeaning, but to no avail until 1978.

Work with long-term heroin addicts is not always a rewarding experience. They are frequently volatile, hostile, and noisy. Addicts are more difficult to work with than most of our other guests (excluding the alcoholics, schizophrenics, or the violent). Some are also persistent thieves. Almost anything and everything that wasn't "nailed down"—office supplies, plants, small furniture, money, typewriters, tape recorders—disappeared regularly until suitable precautions (mostly locking things up) were taken. Many of them smoked at Fort Help, in defiance of our belief that nicotine addiction is objectionable and harmful. Many constantly engaged in "testing" behavior (smoking or making noise) and had to be reminded. For a staff of whom a majority had serious concerns about abuses of authority, this controlling of a few deviants was a difficult task. Sometimes the addicts were blamed for things they couldn't have done. But one of them went so far as to set several fires at the Howard Street building, once destroying the interior of a large room, along with construction supplies. On the one hand, the part of the Howard Street building set aside for methadone services was inadequate. The counseling rooms were unfinished and had the shabbiest of rugs and furniture. A black nurse on the staff appropriately called it "the back of the bus." The methadone staff felt short-changed.

Not everybody approved of methadone. One group, the United States Labor Party, went so far as to plaster posters all over San Francisco, with death threats against Joel and those operating the program, because methadone was a "CIA-Rockefeller plot."

There were three small groups of staff who were also opposed to the methadone program: 1) those who felt the program was unsuccessful, since methadone did not make people drug-free, and that the program absorbed energy that could be more effective elsewhere; 2) those resentful of the better pay for the methadone staff; and 3) those who were unable to deal with the addicts' hostile behavior or staff power struggles. Members of groups 2 and 3 generally overlapped. Although comprising only a fraction of the staff, these malcontents happened to be a considerable portion of core-group leadership at this time. As the homogenization of the counseling staff (including a number of methadone staff working on other problems) had been largely accomplished by the summer of 1973, core group anger turned more and more openly towards the methadone program. As one of our most dedicated staff members put it succinctly, we were a dysfunctional family trying to solve its own unacknowledged internal problems by blaming them on one family member, in this case the methadone program. All would be well if we could just get rid of *them* was the myth.

By the fall of 1973 we were spending two or three hours of core group time every week debating the methadone program. Therefore a staff committee was formed to find a solution. Lothar and four other members found a number of legitimate complaints. Most methadone people indeed worked fewer actual hours than they were paid for. Moreover, collections was allowing sizable amounts of money to remain unaccounted for every week. The counter complaint from the methadone side was that the program itself, staff and clients, was treated unfairly by the staff as a whole. The committee tried to appease both factions: the core group and the staff as a whole were relieved of the endless details while still maintaining control over methadone activities; methadone staff gave up their behind-the-scenes independence in return for a fairer decision-making process. It turned out to be a workable arrangement and led to an era of stability. Many of us wanted all the special programs to coexist, flourish, and cooperate; we would not have liked losing any of our programs. For about a year and a half, the methadone program ran smoothly—democratically self-administered by its staff but receiving Lothar's weekly input as consultant. A physician from Egypt and a psychologist from Australia joined the methadone staff during this period and, with the help of a number of talented home-grown counselors/nurses, stabilized the situation.

In summary, the Antiaddiction and Methadone Maintenance Program operated outside the mainstream of Fort Help activity. Addicts continued to come to Fort Help, where they were never branded as such. Methadone was offered as one option among many, not as a panacea, not even as a preferred mode of help. Other services, including flexible, individualized counseling, were also available to the heroin abusers, but were used infrequently. However, some rift at Fort Help was probably inevitable, given the very divergent life style, minority background, unemployment, and criminal record of most of the addicts when they first arrived.

Equally important, the methadone program was forced to fulfill many state and federal regulations to open and to stay in operation. This unwanted and expensive tie-in with government was necessary but contrary to one of our founding principles. The fact that such a program, still the only private, non-profit, nongovernmental program in California, was allowed to operate at all came from our determination to use methadone as part of the center's comprehensive smorgasbord approach and to fight for the necessary approval. Two third-year medical students from Iowa (representative of the many over the years who came to us for externships, internships, and residencies of a few months to a year) were especially helpful in organizing staff and addicts to gain the necessary government approval referred to earlier in the book.

The Sex and Relationship Program

Our abilities to deal with sexual as well as other problems were suddenly put to the test when we had a sudden influx of guests with sexual concerns, coming to us via Don Chamberlin and his popular radio program, "California Girl." This was a program in which women in the Bay Area could call in to talk, in an uninhibited way, about sex-related topics or problems. Chamberlin invited sex experts, such as Joel, who could contribute professional advice. Joel had taught Sex and Crime at the University of California in Berkeley since 1962, started the San Francisco Health Department's Center for Special Problems' sex program in 1965, and initiated the National Sex Forum for training sex therapists and educators in 1968. He appeared on Chamberlin's show five or six times, over an eighteen-month period, and answered many questions spontaneously on the air; but whenever he perceived a particularly serious situation, he recommended Fort Help's Sex and Relationship Program. Chamberlin liked us and later became a board member.

As a result, inquiries to Fort Help doubled and tripled. We knew in advance that on the morning after one of Joel's appearances on the program the telephones would be ringing continuously with requests for sex and relationship counseling. We had plenty of guests. More importantly, we were able to reach a population that had for the most part eluded us, the middle class. We had long been concerned about this since we believed in nondiscrimination rather than reverse discrimination. Fort Help was not intended to cater exclusively to dropouts, the poor, addicts, or alienated younger people. They were to be welcomed, but not to the exclusion of other segments of the population. A fully functioning, ethical, helping center should attract and serve *everybody*. But this hadn't happened so far.

Most of the people (largely couples) seeking sex counseling, in the nine-county Bay Area that we served, were suburban, usually a combination of working male/dissatisfied housewife; and the socioeconomic range included both managerial and blue collar backgrounds. A common complaint was "we haven't had a good relationship at all," or, "we haven't been able to communicate for a long time." Many responded quickly to our services, but there was also a large dropout rate, more than with other types of guests. The guest load was sometimes staggering, and many of us worked extra hours. Fortunately, at this time, the Fort Help staff was well-balanced between counseling energy and leadership ability. The place was well run by oldtimers on the staff. At the same time, a number of new people who were to fill positions of real leadership joined the staff in 1972, Helen Garvy among them. Helen, in particular, proved to be a responsible person and rapidly worked her way into the center of the decision-making process.

We sorted out the problems between those that could be handled by any counselor and those that needed qualified sex therapists. We helped guests with sexual dysfunction (such as impotence and premature ejaculation), expectational dysfunction (unrealistic expectations, based on misinformation, leading to failure), dysfunction created by physical problems (here we gave medical referrals), and dysfunction rooted in drug abuse. We helped people whose sexual complaints were not dysfunctional but part of larger relationship difficulties. We also helped guests with hetero-homosexual orientation problems.

Many of those calling in for sex counseling were not ready for any kind of intensive work (nor did they need it); what they wanted was accurate, unbiased information. Many otherwise sophisticated adults are still ignorant of basic sexual information, and are concerned about whether their own desires are "normal." Therefore, we instituted large group education and brief counseling sessions. A Fort Help newsletter article, "Marching Through Clitoria," describes our plan for these sessions:

> We are setting up regularly scheduled 'Introduction to Sex Education and Enhancement (S.E.E.)' [sessions]. These are going to start in two weeks. The sessions will be for couples and individuals who are interested in getting some basic information (and perhaps some permission) about sex, as

well as a rundown on Fort Help's programs. The charge will be $20 per couple for at least 1-1/2- to 2-hour sessions. We will need to limit the number of people initially to 50 (because of the construction in the new building) so we will call the people back to set them up for a particular group. I would appreciate that when people call in about sex and relationship questions or problems you could tell them that attending these meetings would be their initial step. Our waiting list is currently 60-75 people/couples—not the 300 that rumor has it, although I must admit it seems really large at times.

Thereafter, we referred new guests to the S.E.E. sessions, and for most, that sufficed. Others were given further screening to see what they needed. Since the general sex therapy program had a small number of staff cotherapists, we had a large waiting list (rare at the center). We referred many couples to other places, such as the sexuality program at the University of California Medical Center. As more of the public became educated, and as more professionals and nonprofessionals began working in the field, the demands for our services decreased. Probably our lack of marketing (except for the free publicity on "California Girl") contributed to the gradual slackening of the demand for the program.

A major aspect of sexual education and treatment was our multimedia approach. We used films and slides, short lectures, exhibits, question-and-answer sessions, and small group discussions as well as massage, body-image work, and similar techniques designed to allow one to relax and to heighten sensual experiences. In the S.E.E. meetings, which a female staff member and Joel conducted once or twice monthly, we tried to debunk the many myths about female and male sexuality. At the same time we encouraged loving relationships and eschewed the trendy focus on casualness and orgasms.

To most of the staff, the idea that the Fort Help ethic *could* include sex with guests never occurred. Two people, however, had what we came to call the "magic penis" concept (not unknown among some male psychiatrists in private practice who are sincerely convinced that sexual counseling without the actual sex act is ineffective). These two proponents on our staff felt that we others were "uptight," and that we should "give them space" to try their more "advanced" techniques. If nudity and massage were acceptable, they reasoned, then drawing an artificial line at intercourse did not make sense. Most of us felt that we could not develop and maintain a reputation as a place for valuable and trusted work if this went on in our midst. One of the two violated the ethic, and we felt that our position as a state-licensed health center could be jeopardized. The resolution was swift and explicit: a hastily called coordinators' meeting, over which Joel presided, expelled the member who had had sexual relations with a guest. We announced a simple, nonnegotiable policy: anyone engaging in sexual activity with any guest (his or her own, or someone else's) would be summarily removed from staff. Once a weak attempt was made by some staff members to eliminate "this authoritarian rule," but it didn't get very far. One of the staff members later did a doctoral dissertation on case studies of women who had been seduced by their therapists; she did not find any involving Fort Help.

In connection with our sex counseling program, another interesting philosophical issue arose in early 1973 at the time of our move from Howard Street to the new quarters. Some staff members objected to using sexual surrogates for a few partnerless guests, even though this was advocated by Masters and Johnson. (Our frame of reference for our sexual therapy was and is a combination of the Kinsey findings, "growth" approaches, and the Masters and Johnson techniques.) Sexual surrogatism did not directly violate the basic policy, although it was not a part of our original program. But the staff was strongly divided on the questions of 1) whether this involved condoning exploitation of the surrogates—largely female—for the benefit of male guests, and 2) whether our reputation as a help center would suffer from these activities. In admirably democratic fashion the skirmishing started with a carefully drawn position paper after many meetings of the sex and relationship program staff and discussion by the entire staff. The position paper was published in the newsletter, which also carried an opposing view. Another view by a staff member suggesting complete permissiveness was also later printed.

At least no one can claim that many people did not put in large amounts of energy doing research on the implications of their favorite arguments. A total of almost six pages of the newsletter are filled with references to discrimination, legality, morality, professional licensing considerations, the reputation of Fort Help, the scarcity of good relationships, therapeutic control, Masters and Johnson, Hartman and Fithian, behaviorism, psychoanalysis, sociology, alcoholism, neo-Freudianism, and finally the fabulous "Phallus in Wonderland" headline from one issue. The arguments were exhaustive (as well as somewhat exhausting) and represented totally divergent value systems. There followed several weeks during which the issue was once more actively discussed by all staff. We called another general meeting, at which the issue was to be settled once and for all. Points and counterpoints on surrogates were summarized in writing, ground rules were set for a written ballot by the entire staff. The results were humorously anticlimactic: the vote to prevent use of surrogates ended in a fifteen-to-fifteen tie. Those who wanted to use surrogates as consultants were able to do so, using the proposed guidelines for such work. This is the closest we came to the time-consuming formalities and legalities of parliamentary procedure.

And there the matter rested. After placing an ad in the *San Francisco Chronicle* for male and female, hetero- and homosexual people to be surrogates, Joel screened and finally selected two female surrogates. The idea had been approved, but it was used very selectively by the staff of the sex program and only at the request of the person seeking help. Only five male guests eventually used the surrogates. There were no problems; those using the surrogates felt that they had been helped. We insisted on an overall ethic that went beyond "professional" standards.

We discovered that in the long run a therapist cannot deal with sexual dysfunctioning on a purely behavioristic level, ignoring the underlying social and psychological difficulties. Eventually, therefore, most of the demands for specific sexual therapy were worked out in the context of relationship counseling, with as much focus on other matters as on sex itself.

Homosexuality

The staff held a progressive position towards homosexuality, both among themselves and in regard to guests. In 1961, Joel had written a statement on nonsickness and equality adopted by the National Homophile Conference, and in 1965 had started the first public program for homosexuals at the Center for Special Problems. At the time of Fort Help's initial program (1970), the American Psychiatric Association still considered homosexuality to be a mental illness that required "treatment." In other words, an individual could not be considered normally functioning unless he or she were heterosexual. And in society at large, the movement of gays "out of the closet" had not really begun.

We considered a person's sexual orientation a matter of personal preference rather than a sign of health or pathology. This was innovative in itself, although, as with most of our professional and human rights achievements, we did not seek or spontaneously receive media recognition for this. Our standard or ethic on homosexuality did not prevent us from working with a homosexual or bisexual guest on their needs. Over a period of years we have had many male and female homosexual counselors on our staff (as well as many heterosexual helpers of both sexes), working with both gay and straight guests on sexual as well as nonsexual issues. Fort Help managed to avoid the reverse segregation and sexism evident at some other institutions. There was no pressuring of people to deal with their anxieties by getting in touch with their homosexual potential, or to be promiscuous, or to be anything else supposedly called for by the media-manufactured sexual revolution. Both homosexual and heterosexual relations between staff and guests were banned.

Feminism

Not surprisingly, the center was also a rallying point for feminist consciousness-raising and women's groups. Women were at least men's equals and in practice more often superior in decision-making powers. The climate encouraged the positive liberation of women's feelings. An early coordinator said:

> I think these groups had a tremendous impact on clients as well as staff-
> —both women and men. It seems to me that the peer respect people held for

each other at Fort Help (at its best) would have been slower to develop and perhaps never would have developed without the very concrete experience of existing in an environment where such attention was paid to the nitty gritty levels of sex and gender roles. There were staff, client and staff/client women's groups from the very early days. For a while Fort Help was almost a women's center, or filled that need. This was important to me and, I suspect, to many others.

Transsexuality

As at the Center for Special Problems, Fort Help also had a gender program for male and female transsexuals. Making life easier for transsexuals was a dream come true for one of our staff, a transsexual who served as a gender counselor. She, like tens of thousands of others in the United States, was born physically a male but from an early age felt psychologically a woman. The combination of first-hand experience and professional training as a psychologist enabled her to offer a unique service to transsexuals. The ultimate goal of most transsexuals is to "cross over," that is, to obtain through plastic surgery the anatomy that matches the gender identification. But transsexuals also need help with legal, cosmetic, and employment problems, as well as psychological counseling. We counseled an average of twenty to thirty such clients at a given time.

A comprehensive program of psychological and social evaluation, counseling, and hormone treatment was made available to transsexuals at Fort Help for whatever they were able to pay. The counseling and hormone treatments last about two years, a period of time that insures against mistakes in the subsequent decision to seek surgery. We were fortunate in having available as a consultant and occasional guest lecturer, **Dr. Harry Benjamin**, the leading authority on this subject.

Violence Prevention Program

For most adult Americans, violence is an important concern of our age. The standard approaches of politicians and legislators have been talking, promising, issuing press releases, appointing committees for more studies, or calling for more police. The sensationalizing of and preoccupation with violence by the media have also exacerbated the situation. Crime pays; violence increases in the home, on the streets, and on television; there is massive neglect of victims, their families and friends. No one program or one person will solve, curb, or prevent all violence. But the Violence Prevention Service at Fort Help had hopes of making a dent in it. Fort Help inherited a concern about crime and violence from the earlier San Francisco Health Department's programs and its Jail Rehabilitation Branch. Our new and much needed project drew on our collective experience, but was entirely separate in staffing and financing when it began in 1977. None of the limited funds of the center were diverted, but this project did use one room at the Fort.

We provided services to three particular groups of people: those contemplating or perpetrating violence (murder, assault, rape, spouse or child abuse, sexual sadism, drunk driving); victims of violence; friends and family members of the victims and of the violent. For the most part too little was or is now available to help these people, but we tried to avoid duplicating good services already in existence, such as Women Against Rape and Suicide Prevention. The first group to be served was partially analagous to those who seek help by telephone for suicidal thoughts or intentions. However, some who have already carried out violent acts will call us for help to prevent recurrences or to deal with guilt and anxiety. The second group who need this new form of help is probably much larger: the direct victims of violence. The family and friends of the victims, including those who are left to suffer after the sudden death of a family member from homicide or suicide, are also many. This includes children old enough to benefit from telephone help.

Like the Fort Help number (864-HELP) the telephone number for Violence Prevention was carefully chosen for easy recall: 86-HUMAN. The telephone help was provided by a specially trained and carefully selected staff. The services included social and psychological counseling; catharsis, a safe and trusted way to voice outrage, anger, fear, and guilt; advice on police and legal assistance, victim compensation programs, and other sources of practical, relevant help; and when indicated, referral for on-going hospital or out-patient treatment, sometimes at Fort Help. But, unfortunately, we did not receive enough calls to justify continuing the hotline or the time commitment of the carefully trained and unpaid staff. Now we maintain only the education and consulting programs, except for receiving a few telephone calls per week for help.

Breathe Free (Stop Smoking) Program

The staff, with a few notable exceptions, never got interested enough about the problems of death, disability, pollution, and property damage resulting from tobacco smoking. However, they strongly supported the nonsmoking ethic at Fort Help (Appendix D). Joel established large-group education and treatment sessions once a month, when there were enough people signed up (by telephone) to justify it. His feeling was that our two biggest drug problems, alcohol and tobacco, deserve as much attention as heroin, that drug programs should work on all mind-altering drugs. Only Helen, Meg, and a few others shared that commitment. We mailed out a variety of educational materials to those who wrote or telephoned. We also mailed sex and drug articles, charts, and pamphlets, as part of the Fort's public education and prevention activities, usually without charge. Sometimes one or two staff members helped with the program, and a few others were given training through it. We gave away buttons saying "Yes I Do Mind—Please don't smoke anything in public."

The Breathe Free group sessions included a short, amusing, and honest antismoking film; a concise lecture on the history of tobacco use, the reasons why people smoke, and the effects on both smokers and nonsmokers; questions and discussion; and most importantly, a variety of techniques for stopping, from deep-breathing exercises and behavior modification to immunization against advertising of cigarettes (merchandising death) and peer pressure. The Breathe Free sessions, like the S.E.E. program, attracted mostly middle- and upper-income people. So we charged a moderate fee but characteristically also allowed in those who could not pay. We have now no direct services for smokers.

Slim Chance (Overeaters) Program

Many staff members worked on this program over the years (a few after first coming to us for help with obesity), after Joel got it started, feeling this was another pervasive, inadequately dealt with *social* problem. Usually help was given through a time-limited (four to six 1-1/2- to 2-hour sessions) group of ten to fifteen people, and co-led by a male and a female staff member. We began by explaining the possible social and psychological reasons for overeating, having each person describe his or her eating pattern, trying to immunize him or her against peer, family, and advertising pressures to overeat, and training him or her in a wide range of helping techniques. Body image work (exploring feelings about different parts of the body when standing unclothed before a mirror, in private); a telephone buddy to call when the group member felt the urge to overeat; exercise; group discussion and support, behavior modification techniques; and written suggestions (Appendix E) were used in tandem. As with other programs (except selective use of methadone and hormones) we used neither drugs nor long-term psychotherapy. There was and is a sliding fee scale.

OPERATIONS

Rewards and stipends

One of the most significant powers at the center of any operation is the authority to determine rewards. Potentially we can categorize these rewards as follows: 1) satisfaction in doing a good and socially valuable job; 2) freedom to be innovative; 3) freedom from interference; 4) status and position; and 5) money. At Fort Help, social significance, innovation, and lack of interference were consistently available. An avoidance of status and position, however, was fundamental to the ethic of Fort Help. Money, of course, was always in very limited supply.

Everyone's contribution of time was considered of equal value. The time issue also spilled over, naturally and expectedly, into money matters, specifically the minimal stipends paid to some of the staff. This was always a difficult situation; there was little income but many people wanting some small monetary compensation. In the beginning only the coordinators (except for Joel) received modest stipends (usually around $100 weekly), since they were spending most of their time at Fort Help. As more funds became available, other key staff members who carried heavy counseling schedules in addition to other work were also salaried at $50 to $75 weekly. In the first year or two some eight people on staff (exclusive of the methadone program, where most staff members had higher salaries) had minimal income while the other thirty or so received no income from the Fort. Each year the proportion of staff members receiving payment increased, although people were expected to show their ability and commitment for some months before going on stipend. Criteria for stipends were officially established in 1972, with all generalists eligible to apply (Appendix F). We rewarded those making the greatest contribution to keeping the center functioning, as well as those people in greatest financial need.

Concentrating the limited, available funds on keeping key people was later openly rejected by a staff majority. The policy of varying salaries according to what the staff member said he or she needed was also eventually vetoed. Later almost everybody who wanted a stipend was granted one (for identical amounts). This is in some ways fair, but fails to differentiate between the very competent and beginners, among varying needs, and to deal with the practical realities of keeping people with high earning potential. Philosophical points can be made on both sides of the question. But the pragmatic outcome was that, when we opted in favor of the equal system, we lost the majority of the most experienced staff.

Staff Profile

The *average* level of staff competence in 1976 (and 1980) was probably the equivalent of what was reached during 1972, when emphasis was on quality of services rather than self-determination. The similarity can be deceiving. At the earlier date, with a large staff and much turnover, we had a considerable number of really first-class generalists and a fair number of average ones. Four years later, there were fewer good ones, a small number well on their way to being good, and a large number who were adequate but not outstanding. Even though the "average" skills of a staff member, therefore, comes out the same in both instances, Lothar feels the earlier staff profile was preferable, since the less capable ones dropped out and there were more people on staff to whom one could refer difficult cases with confidence.

In regard to professional degrees, less than ten M.D.s and ten Ph.D.s came to us, much to Joel's disappointment. He wanted a multibackground staff based on competence rather than credentials, but some of whom would have the credentials as an important resource anyway. It was not that we failed to attract many capable people. The problem was that too many of them left after six months or a year, although a surprising number stayed on longer out of a sense of dedication.

Our struggle to establish standards was one of the key problems for many years. Limits based on competence must be recognized and respected. While being totally open to new staff members, we stressed the apprenticeship concept concomitantly. A core staff of people who know what they are doing must be encouraged and kept as intact as possible. At Fort Help the energy of these valuable people often went unrewarded, as they had to underpin the work of unskilled staff who sometimes refused to recognize their own limitations.

There were occasions in which being part of the Fort Help staff proved overwhelming for some. The general atmosphere was to encourage innovation. Since there was no authoritarian or hierarchical supervisor to whom one was responsible, and since there was so much to be done, a helper found it hard to say to the whole staff, "I'm having some problems, can you take care of my schedule for a couple of weeks?" Thus in a few instances people who were not particularly adept at self-regulation drove themselves to the point of collapse.

Training

Training was and is an ongoing concern. In the earlier stages of Fort Help, most of the staff had no formal background in behavioral science or medicine. The basic training plan included lectures, role playing, group discussion, outside seminars, and apprenticeship. This was soon augmented by some special training sessions for the entire staff, including several on sexuality and one on communication skills. Outside resource people participated, along with Joel, in a fascinating day-long psychodrama session directed by Lewis Yablonsky, one of the leading experts in that field. This session was videotaped and later shown on KQED-TV, San Francisco's public television station. Dr. Harry Benjamin and Ed Brecher, a prominent writer on the subject, gave unforgettable, warmly human lectures on sex. We presented authoritative sessions on primal screaming, gestalt therapy, and poetry therapy. We held many workshops to gain competency in our smorgasbord approach. Joel led a three-hour panel discussion on depression and suicide. Lothar held sessions on bioenergetic therapy and on family therapy.

It proved difficult to maintain a consistent staff training and supervision program. Originally, these sessions were conducted on Saturdays. As staff members became reluctant to give up part of their weekends, we held training sessions more sporadically. Then we established a formal training program, which was mandatory for all new staff. By 1976 this formal training had become quite sophisticated and covered the basic principles needed by a beginning helper; we taught this course over a six- or seven-week period. At the same time we decided not to take on new staff singly but rather in groups of six to seven, two or three times a year, so the whole training and orientation procedure could be better controlled.

Funding

The main question some readers will have is how to obtain funds if the most popular source, government, is eliminated in advance by creative and ethical choice. Even if most people's time is freely contributed temporarily and a few permanently, there are still rent, building materials, supplies, and telephones to consider. The initial 1970 statement in this regard was simple and direct: we will be financed through guest fees, mostly from middle- and upper-income people, supplemented by some tax-exempt donations, foundation grants, special fund raising projects, low overhead (administrative and rental costs), and volunteer services.

This sounds simpler than it really was. Fees were always considered to be the prime source of cash income; but they have an unpleasant attribute in that one has to *ask* for them individually. This created two immediate problems. In the first place there was a considerable contingent of staff who felt that helping services are a *right* and that it is "immoral" to ask for payment. The more doctrinaire they were, the less inclined they were to compromise their "ideals," even in the face of the need for money to pay the rent to maintain facilities where they could provide free services. And some of them, inconsistently, were even among the most insistent that *they* should be paid for their services since they "needed the bread," though they did not want to concern themselves with collecting it. Luckily most of the staff had a better understanding of economics and of idealism; otherwise the Fort Help experiment might not have succeeded.

The second problem was more subtle. *Asking* for money is difficult to do. In the first place, if you are not sure how much your services are really worth, how comfortable are you going to be asking a guest to pay $20 to $30 for an hour or more of your time? In the second place, many professionals in the social and mental health fields are not used to dealing with money at all. This is handled by a secretary, billing clerk, or nurse at the desk. "Haggling" is "unprofessional"; money is an embarrassing subject to many. It is incongruous to be quite comfortable discussing the most intimate details of a person's sex life with him or her and to be uncomfortable about the particulars of setting a fee, but it happens even in a money-oriented society. Additionally, from the beginning we gave considerable help by telephone and none of this was paid for, although Joel suggested that in selected instances people be asked to send in money or at least that the more distant calls be made collect. (As part of our revolutionary approach to paperwork and to use of time, we have never sent bills.)

From the very beginning, we had seminars for the staff on how to deal with money issues, and most people learned. However, it seemed that most of the guests who came to Fort Help for assistance were close to being broke, or claimed they were. Dealing with the guest who said he or she had no money to pay for the counseling, but who was spending significant amounts each week for alcohol, heroin, tobacco, and taxis, was a recurrent problem. At one time a staff member refused to work with a guest who wanted advice on his potency problems but declined to pay "because then I wouldn't have enough money to take the chicks out and fuck 'em!" The middle class people who could afford moderate fees, if asked, were at first few. During 1972, Lothar collected a total of $4,700 for Fort Help from the people he was helping, averaging approximately $10 per session. This represented about twenty-five percent of the center's cash fee income that year, even though he was only one of perhaps twenty generalist problem-solvers on the staff at the time.

In spite of, or perhaps because of, our high ideals, Fort Help might have had to close its doors during its second year of operation had it not been for foundation money. The modest costs of the early months had been borne by Joel, out of his irregular income from lecturing, consulting, and writing. Rent (even at a low $300 per month), telephone and supply bills started piling up, and some of the staff needed income to meet their personal needs. In the spring of 1971, when things were beginning to get critical, Joel and Meg persuaded the San Francisco Foundation to give us a grant of $25,000, payable in four quarterly installments, as seed money. For the first time, some key people were able to take home $50 or $100 a week for the services rendered at Fort Help, and some who would not otherwise have been able to stay could continue.

The San Francisco Foundation extended the $25,000 grant the following year, and then gave a final third-year grant of $15,000, ending in the fall of 1973. All of this was allocated for staff stipends, none for administration or equipment. Our success in this respect encouraged us to apply to other foundations for support, for it was obvious that this was a good potential source of large-scale funds. But we were unsuccessful.

At meetings we talked of the strings attached to all outside funding, with foundations requiring the fewest compromises. Thinking that we had shown a lack of initiative and innovation in fund raising, we brainstormed for ideas. One thing we needed and got was people to make telephone calls or visits for free materials such as paint, fabric for curtains, and carpets. Much of what we did was born in desperation. Joel managed (as he did from time to time) to obtain contributions in the $500-$1,000 range from such board members as Arthur Rock and Cecil Whitebone. An art auction, a dress sale by board member Alvin Duskin, the closing Fillmore West concert of Creedence Clearwater, and similar events raised a few hundred dollars here and there. In terms of the overall cash needs, these were "drops in the bucket."

Meg Holmberg, M., and L. carried out a concentrated campaign to get major foundation support. Most foundations did not even reply to our requests, and the ones that did gave us a negative response. The failure considerably dampened our spirits. Perhaps our failure was due to our lack of public stature or because our applications were possibly amateurish. We honestly stressed things which, though dear to us, were probably dubious to foundation people: Not having administrators is great, but who is then going to be responsible? Having low-paid staff is laudable, but where are the "experts"? We were communicating in a language foundation administrators didn't understand, and the fact that we were sincere, dedicated, and already successful in the best sense didn't help. Fund raising is a conservative field, and we probably came across as revolutionary.

Our Own Space

Our systematic search for new and better quarters, and the resulting many discussions, refined what we wanted and needed. We summarized in October 1972:

> Here's where we stand in our building search. There is nothing new and exciting to report. We decided several months ago that we really liked the building at 3265 16th Street (between Dolores and Guerrero). It is 13,000 square feet (we now have 4,600) on two floors. It is mainly open space and will require a fair amount of work to be divided up into the small areas that we need. It has few windows (except a plate glass front downstairs and some windows upstairs that can be unboarded). It is in good condition, located close to transportation. We would need a $40,000 down payment, and we don't have it.

> We have one other possible building—the (former) Hare Krishna temple on Valencia Street between 15th and 16th Streets. It has 8,000 square feet on two floors plus a small basement part. It is divided into a bunch of large and small rooms, has lots of windows, is brightly painted and ready to use as it is. It is close to busses, but the location is much less 'respectable' than the 16th Street building (location seems to be its major disadvantage). It is for sale for about $85,000 and would probably require a $25,000 down payment.

Explorations with foundations were unsuccessful, and we had no collateral for a bank loan. Helen Garvy summarized:

> Our requirements on location: central, near public transportation, parking available; hopefully neutral enough neighborhood so most will come there; on cost: at this point we're considering buying or renting and we can probably afford $900-$1,000 a month, either in rent or mortgage payments and taxes; on layout: can be adapted to our needs without too much immediate work (like no big open warehouse) or can be warehouse with some divisions already, office space, or a set of apartments, 7,000 to 10,000 square feet would be ideal; on legal requirements: zoned for F-2 occupancy which means few restrictions, can be in any commercial or manufacturing zone but we can

also be in R-4 and R-5 (residential) zones, although would need a public hearing first, which it could be hard to win.

Helen was well informed about buildings and construction (as well as social change and organizations). Her tenacity in this respect kept us from standing "out in the rain" on Tenth Street one day with no place to go. Finally, the November 17 newsletter reported the success of the building search group of Helen, Meg, and Joel. The staff met and after discussion, a vote was taken with Eleventh Street (our current location) winning eleven to two. There was a sense of excitement and a resurgence of optimism. Collectively, we had solved still another difficult problem. In-depth study and discussion took place about just what kind of space to create for ourselves in the much larger area that would be available to us, how to use it, and what priorities to set. (See Appendix G.)

The outlines of the actual construction on both floors were readily approved. What happened on the ground floor stayed very close to the committee decisions and to the plans, as agreed upon. We recommended a more functional telephone room, and both a "quiet" living room and a "noisier" one for guests who wanted to do more than just sit and wait. Establishing the telephone area within a large, otherwise unwalled staff room turned out to be not too happy a choice, but the main living room is large and graceful. The upstairs rooms did not fare so well at first, but over the next year they were individually decorated and redesigned by staff members although they continued to be shared on a sign-up basis. The area for former heroin addicts on the methadone program was left unfinished for some months, reflective of tensions among some of our programs that were to produce intermittent problems over the years.

Being by choice a low-budget place not accepting government funds, we were in need of basic furnishings, so an appeal was made to selected individuals for help. In 1973 we asked for equipment and furnishings: lamps, sofas, bookcases, cabinets, typewriters, tape recorders, light bulbs, and, of course, money. Many responded. John Connelly, a Northern California businessman, who later became a member of our board of directors, happened to be demolishing a building he owned on Sansome Street, and generously told us we could remove anything we wanted from the inside of the building. We took carpets, walnut wall paneling, a dozen walnut doors, construction materials, thousands of pieces of acoustical tile, bathroom fixtures, hardwood counters, and lamps. Our need for actual building materials, other than two-by-fours and sheet rock, was thus held to a minimum, and we saved thousands of dollars.

There were several "construction weekends" when large numbers of staff members came to help build our new surroundings. However, Helen and a small crew of volunteers ended up doing the most of the work. On "opening day" at 169 Eleventh Street, some of the doors were not yet hung, floors were not yet finished, and not all the ceiling tiles had yet been installed in the phone room. We prevailed upon a friend, Robert Kantor, an attorney who likewise later joined the board of directors, to arrange a contribution in a roundabout way: a donation of $1,000 was made to the Delancey Street organization with the understanding that one of their construction crews would help finish the Fort Help facility. Instead of an experienced construction crew, however, they sent some trainees who insisted on being paid an experienced carpenter's wage of $7 per hour. They did not get very much done; our $1,000 was used up rapidly; but at least the doors were hung and half the ceiling tile was put in place.

Some plants died because people would walk right by them all day without ever thinking of watering them, until one or two people took on the task. This also happened with other things that properly took second place to direct human services, but also needed to be done. Until 1976, there was usually some aspect of the environment that was unfinished or being redone for variety or improvement.

Both group energy and aesthetic concern waxed and waned over the years, but eventually old furnishings were replaced, walls repainted, the floors were cleaned, and the initial concept of a bright, futuristic design was realized. Today it looks like a place one wants to go to and work in.

Chapter 4
CRISES WEATHERED

I remember my youth and the feeling that will never come back. . .the feeling that I could outlast the sea, the earth, and all men. —Joseph Conrad

Developing a new organization is a creative opportunity in life, as well as a major challenge. We start with an age of innocence and confidence, assuming that the strength of our ideals and abilities will carry the day. Any later development depends on how, and whether, we are able to come to grips with the intrusion of harsh realities. Such was our experience at Fort Help, where the methadone program's financial crisis and the breakdown of participatory democracy among the staff were two of our harsh realities. Soon there were other intrusions. Trade-offs and compromises occurred at Fort Help. Parts of the dream never became reality.

RADICALISM

One crisis arose gradually out of several sources. Experience slowly taught us what was feasible and what wasn't, but some staff rhetoric remained the same. The more radical people on staff were unwilling to accept the gradual reduction in participatory democracy demanded by actual work performance. They demanded frequent meetings, they were the most verbal and loudest ones at the meetings, they stayed after others became disgusted and left, and they tended to dominate some decisions. In practice it seemed that those who were doing the least helping of guests had the most time to spend in meetings.

The system that had evolved to deal with this was one of delegated powers. General meetings of the staff were held at intervals ranging from monthly to bimonthly to deal with general policy and to elect the coordinators. The coordinators made the day-to-day operating decisions, with at least two of the four taking part. This made the organization fairly stable, but it also offended those who resisted any kind of structure, even if it was needed to insure quality and continuity of services. During the early fall of 1971, tension between the two factions became ever greater, especially as it was aggravated by another anxiety-producing process.

In October 1971, when we least needed it, a figurative bomb exploded in our faces and all but brought Fort Help to a close. We had been aware that all was not well with the organization and finances of the antiaddiction program but no one was prepared for what we learned (See Appendix H). Not only was the methadone program deeply in debt but the whole center was practically bankrupt because of this one special program.

Many of the people on the Antiaddiction and Methadone Maintenance Program came to us as street addicts. They somehow were able to find hundreds of dollars a *day* to support their habit, so it had seemed reasonable to expect them to pay $20 per *week* for our services. But many of them had no job skills and these methods they had used to support their habit previously were not legal. They were depressed, had police records, or simply didn't want to work, so that raising legitimately even a small fraction of what they had previously been paying for drugs was difficult. They had fallen behind in their payments, and a kindly staff member (who, like a number of others, had difficulty asking guests for money) had let some of them pile up debts of hundreds of dollars. Joel had been abroad at the time; other coordinators had shown themselves to be inept or careless at financial management. Suddenly, we found ourselves with about $15,000 of accounts receivable and large bills owed to the laboratory doing the federal- and state-required urine testing for drugs. The lab threatened to cut us off unless they were paid promptly.

At this point, some of the more radical staff members decided to manipulate the situation in their own favor. They had been trying to turn us into a rap (encounter group) center. A rap center could not possibly provide the services for which Fort Help was organized. The majority of staff members, especially the counseling staff, wanted the necessary existing structure to go with the work we were doing. The more radical people had gone along grudgingly with these developments in the beginning, however. Now they were being faced with reassessment, and the small number of radicals had rejected the idea that anyone had to be assessed or qualified to do anything. For them, capability was "bureaucratic bullshit." If you wanted to do primal therapy or hypnosis you should be free to do so.

These radicals (extremists, pseudo-revolutionaries as we thought of them) now chose to ally themselves with those methadone guests who had not paid their bills (and didn't want to pay). They claimed that the fault lay with "the system" for "victimizing" these guests. In order to terminate the "exploitation" they railed against, they believed that all distinctions between staff and guests should be abolished. The irony was that we had already eliminated many traditional practices. Our only distinction here was between ex-heroin addicts coming for help and nonaddicts providing help.

Some time previously we decided that our methadone guests should be given regular access to staff meetings by electing ten of their own number as nonvoting representatives to speak for them. We had hoped this would regularize a process that was evident anyway, informally attending staff meetings to listen and speak. At the October staff meeting, as the minutes show, an attempt was now made to take control by giving votes to these ten guest representatives. It was barely defeated. At the time, the center was run by the three elected coordinators, with Joel ex-officio, rather than by the general staff meeting. Since the coordinators themselves were chosen at these staff meetings, they could easily have been replaced by radicals unable to meet the financial crisis with anything other than angry rhetoric and wishful thinking. This irresponsible proposal to let the very guests whose failure to pay their bills had precipitated our crisis now sabotaged our efforts to pull out of our financial problem. The fact that it had almost succeeded made many of us despair of finding a solution to the problem under the current structure.

At Lothar's initiative, the generalists—those upon whose performance the center depended most heavily—held a private meeting. We saw a year-and-a-half of hard work going down the drain; the old joke about the "inmates taking over the asylum" was literally about to come true. Our decision at the meeting was to turn to Joel for direction, since we seemed unable to solve the problem. It is characteristic of him that he resisted doing this; we had to convince him we could not continue serving at the center under the present chaotic circumstances. It is equally characteristic of him that he responded quickly. He called a special meeting for October 30, and acted to resolve the crisis. During this time, one of the addict guests went to the *San Francisco Chronicle*, resulting in problems being reported publicly, thus adding to the pressure. In addition, two lists of staff problems and/or grievances relative to the same matter were also being circulated through the center.

Almost sixty staff members attended the October 30th meeting. We spent most of the afternoon in discussion: More structure or less structure? Tighter assessment or open assessment? What should we do about the financial crisis? Was the meeting valid, since it had not been called by the staff as a whole? Despite encouraging full participation and seeking workable, concrete solutions, none was forthcoming. Finally, Joel acted. He announced that instead of the single, tough administrator a number of people had called for, the position of the coordinators would be strengthened. However, since our system of participatory democracy was producing dissension, keeping us from attending to the real goals of the center, the system would have to be drastically changed. He reminded everyone that he had invited them to be on the staff. His decision—he would again invite those whom he wished to continue serving, after individual consultation. He would temporarily take personal responsibility and accountability for major decisions, and would appoint new coordinators to supervise day-to-day operations. After no more than sixty days, all these changes would be reevaluated and hopefully replaced with a better system of self-government.

He had acted much more decisively and more dramatically than most of the staff had expected. In large measure, he had the consent of the governed. Over the next few weeks the staff shrank by almost a third, as the radicals and their supporters left. There was no noticeable reduction in services, curiously. We felt justified in bypassing a process that had become self-destructive. Fort Help needed to be rescued and returned to its main mission. We could either have provided services to people crying out for help or have been totally protective of some unstable staff. We were not willing to make staff process a priority over services to the community.

THIRD-PARTY PAYMENTS

In mid-1972 the staff made a fateful decision to get involved with Medi-Cal, for third-party payments. Joel had objected even to this indirect involvement with government bureaucracy, but went along with the majority at the time. Our newsletter carried an announcement of this event:

> After months of negotiating, Fort Help now has an official Medi-Cal number, allowing us to work with guests who qualify for that program and wish to use it to reciprocate for the help received. This means the state will reimburse us for professional services rendered. Two things can be done to expedite matters: 1) all staff members are asked to compile a list of their clients who are eligible for Medi-Cal and give the information to Meg Holmberg; 2) ask your clients to save their 'stickers' for possible use at Fort Help. These stickers, or labels, are provided to Medi-Cal eligible persons for identification/billing purposes. We will need to turn in these stickers as services are rendered. There is a good chance that the work anyone on the staff or at least those who have had a year or more of graduate school in a psychology-medical-related field, and who is currently being supervised by a person with a professional license will be acceptable. We are waiting for Health Care Services in Sacramento for a ruling on this. Medi-Cal can also be used to reimburse us for counseling provided to those on the methadone program.

From that point on, Medi-Cal fees became a growing percentage of Fort Help income, both for general counseling purposes and for those on the methadone program. Also, both the number and dollar amount of *cash* (or check) fee payments constantly increased as well. Our guest load continued to be weighted towards a high percentage of those unable or unwilling to pay for their services. In such instances, when they were eligible, we took Medi-Cal stickers. This was always a mixed blessing. While it provided necessary funds, an over-dependency develops if a large percentage of a program's income comes from a single source. (That this was more psychological than real was shown after we had stopped Medi-Cal in 1976. We had only brief financial uncertainty, without crisis, and emerged with a stronger financial situation than ever.)

But we had many problems with both the California Health Department and Blue Cross bureaucracies, who were confused, inefficient, and unable to give us clear answers to our questions. Joel allowed his name and medical license to be used under our ethic of democratic decision-making, with the clear understanding that this would be done only as long as it was allowed by the law and regulations. In 1976, there were rumors of Medi-Cal rule changes, followed by several months of unpaid claims without explanation. A total of $80,000 was due to us. Joel arranged a meeting in Sacramento with the former deputy director of the California Department of Public Health and with the state officials to explore these issues. Although they were complimentary of our Fort Help operations, they were evasive and ambiguous about the current regulations. Joel therefore decided immediately to stop all use of his license for Medi-Cal, in order that there would be no trouble for the Fort.

When we asked about the delay of payments to us, Blue Cross responded with requests for additional diagnoses. We provided these, but still did not receive our payment. Even at the time of writing, nearly five years later, we have never been paid. It would seem that, without notice or due process, the state has informally but officially "fined us" that amount.

A few days before Christmas 1977, without any notices or receipt of charges from the state, there suddenly appeared headline stories on television and radio, and in the major newspapers, that Fort Help and Joel had been involved in Medi-Cal fraud. *Not a single reporter had talked to Joel or any other staff member*, or bothered to look up the easily available facts. A press release sent by the state health department contained a series of false charges against Joel, which were later dropped. We later learned that never before had the department issued a press release about charges, or even convictions, against a doctor. The relatively minor issue behind the formal charges, when they were finally received, was whether the counseling services provided by nonmedical staff members were still reimbursable by the state, as had been the case when the center staff signed up with Medi-Cal. Leaving aside the ample evidence that helping ability doesn't reside solely with doctors, it seems that at some point the regulations had been changed for private, nonprofit programs, but not for government programs which could bill for services provided by a wide range of staff.

Then followed an interminable, expensive administrative and judicial process of seeking justice and vindication. Despite a law requiring a hearing within forty-five days, we waited fourteen months for an administrative hearing. The State Board of Medical Quality Assurance had refused Joel's request for a prompt hearing before a panel of doctors, as was permitted with most physicians, including those guilty of malpractice, drug pushing, and sexual indiscretions. The center, forced to obtain legal help, was fortunate to get attorney Charles O'Brien, one of our board members and former chief deputy attorney general. Finally, we had a five-day hearing before a hearing officer (a state employee in regular contact with the prosecutor from the state attorney general's office). All witnesses admitted that Joel had never personally received or asked for money from Medi-Cal for himself; that the regulations were voluminous and confusing; and that no other physician had been attacked in this manner. Adding to the strain of the hearing was the daily harassment in the hearing room by the extremist United States Labor Party, which was daily libeling us as "mass murderers." The judge eliminated cross-examination of the state administrator testifying for the prosecution. He concluded the hearing by expressing hopes that Joel would stay in public life. Next was the agony of a two-month wait for the judicial decision. It came; it was that Joel was altruistic, honest, had not lied or profited, and had authorized use of his name only where legal. One would think this would lead to an unequivocal decision of acquittal, but instead there was a technical finding of unprofessional conduct (not fraud) for allowing his name and license to be used by the staff, and a suspended sentence of three months loss of license. The center as a whole was dropped from the proceeding by mutual agreement, and suffered no penalty apart from the apparent "fine" of the $80,000 owed by Medi-Cal.

In 1979, Joel appealed this decision, starting with the Superior Court of San Francisco. We had another frustrating and stressful wait of fourteen months for a nondecision, an opinion affirming the ruling of the administrative judge. No reasons were given, no indication that either the evidence or the law had been studied. He appealed again. At the time of writing, the matter rests with a three-judge state Court of Appeals—three years since the false charges and libel, and four years since the center stopped using Medi-Cal.

A COMMUNITY AMONG OURSELVES

In this atmosphere, two events again changed the overall course of Fort Help. An experienced Esalen group leader held a marathon staff encounter. With skillful gestalt techniques he managed slowly to crystallize a real concern: Some of the staff were primarily interested in creating a community among themselves with only a secondary aim of providing services, while others were dedicated to running an alternative health services organization to which staff gratifications were secondary.

The issue was, naturally, much more complex. The community priority was in many respects a truly communal one: people wanted to spend as much of their time and energy as possible together, to concentrate on meeting each other's personal needs. Out of this harmonious flow—"we want to create a community so perfect that *everyone* will want to belong to it"—things would somehow happen to take care of the center's guests. Working and living would be integrated. These visionaries were willing to sacrifice other gratifications, such as financial ones, for the achievement of their idea of happiness.

The people on the other side of the issue were pragmatic as well as idealistic. In their estimation, the fact that a more alternative organization enabled us to work with guests in a nonjudgmental fashion, while avoiding the constant restrictions of a traditional bureaucracy, was a remarkable achievement. Who needed more, especially at the cost of dissension? Moreover, this part of the staff had decided to take care of its needs by treating Fort Help as a great place to work but not to live and breathe. And since paying bills was an unavoidable part of life on the outside, some minimal remuneration would be needed.

The first group had been the one dominating Fort Help leadership. They confidently expected a majority of the staff, most of whom didn't choose to attend staff meetings, to show their approval. The results were totally unexpected and dismaying to some: less than twenty percent of those present opted for the community concept as a primary goal; the others held firm to the idea that services to guests came first. Without much fanfare, and unfortunately, several members of the first group gradually drifted away from the center over a period of several months.

Chapter 5

FORT HELP AND ITS FORERUNNERS TODAY

Everything which is now regarded as very ancient was once new, and what we are defending today by precedent will by and by be a precedent itself. —Tacitus

The climate that had resulted in the birth of Fort Help had several facets: the broad social changes and, sometimes, progress of the 1960s; the growing awareness that many of our institutions and leaders were incompetent and corrupt; the realization that there was much selfishness, alienation, and depersonalization all around us. The so-called counterculture turned out to be not strong enough, let alone organized, to break down the core institutions of traditional society. Too many reformers expected immediate success without really concerted effort. Many saw America as the walls of Jericho. When the walls didn't crumble at the blowing of the trumpet, when America wasn't "greened" overnight, people either picked up their instruments and went home to conventional work, or, embittered, went underground into those dark catacombs of the mind where bombs are fashioned out of what had been love.

While Fort Help has not fulfilled all of its ambitious expectations, so far, and has not achieved all the levels of excellence of which it might have been capable—considering the quality of many of the staff and its high principles —it is today still a dynamic and original organization.

Clearly the most striking and most objective thing to be said about Fort Help today is that it is there. It has survived for ten long and sometimes difficult years, generally hale and hearty, somewhat bloodied but unbowed, and with its major ideals and innovations intact. It is continuing on into the future.

The center continues to provide help and hope to thousands of people with a great diversity of problems, backgrounds, and ages. It continues to be an idealistically ambitious, complex, and comprehensive program operating totally without government funding or subsidy, and without public relations or media support. At approximately one-tenth of the cost of a comparable government program, a nonhierarchical, nonbureaucratic organization is being maintained with equality and leadership for women and men, younger and older, homosexuals and heterosexuals, paid and unpaid, with and without professional degrees (paraprofessional, nonprofessional). There is still flexible scheduling of hours and days; part-time work for those who wish to combine a helping career with other important things such as parenthood or authorship of books; training and apprenticeships for new careers; an informal and attractive ("living room") physical environment; a nonmedical, nonpsychiatric, and nonsickness model of help; an eclectic, smorgasbord helping-approach with flexibility, informality, and freedom of choice; extensive telephone help; and ethical standards emphasizing altruism, relevance, and an absence of exploitation or violence, including not smoking in the presence of others.

R., one of the current leaders of the center, in a recent letter to friends, guests, and former staff of Fort Help, recalls the center's "long history of service to thousands in the community with low-cost counseling services and a private, independent methadone maintenance program, while giving a chance to hundreds of staff to train, learn, and earn in an alternative, nonbureaucratic setting; a wide range of high quality approaches to counseling/therapy free of cold clinical procedures and settings; and a model of nongovernmental social service and cooperative administration."

Although we usually don't think about it, no generally accepted system or technique of evaluation exists for programs or organizations, public or private, profit-making or nonprofit. With extremely rare exceptions, governmental and government-subsidized organizations continue indefinitely, and businesses continue as long as they make a profit or at least break even. Often neither quantitative nor qualitative organizational or individual standards are applied to determine performance, let alone excellence. As part of the progressive debasement of language, an image of greatness (often self-engendered through one or another form of advertising) substitutes for the reality of mediocrity or exploitation. To insure that we accurately summarized the present state of Fort Help, we held conversations with a representative sample of currently active staff members as well as with a few who were no longer active but had been deeply involved for many years. The oldest active staff member, M., now age seventy-two, has been on the staff eight years. By coincidence, she began the same day as one of our youngest staff members, then age eighteen. She was also part of our only mother-son staff team. Her work and the place itself continue to be significant to her but she (and others, including the

authors) misses the sense of excitement and pioneering that was present perhaps as long ago as 1975. Others speak of "the Fort" as their most significant
life experience, an all-encompassing one of great vitality.

There are now thirty-seven staff members, thirty in what is now called the
counseling program, and seven in the semiautonomous methadone maintenance program. Over the years many staff members have worked in both of
these now-separate programs. One staff member, I., works in both and also is
the coordinator-nurse (program director in state and federal terminology) of
the methadone program. Most of the staff are part-time, usually twenty hours
per week with some working ten hours and a few twenty-five hours or more.
They now receive a stipend in the general program of $350/month gross for a
twenty-hour week and half that amount for a ten-hour week. There are still no
administrative or medical/psychiatric titles or hierarchies, and all those receiving pay are paid the same amount for the same number of hours. The methadone staff is mostly full-time, with yearly salaries ranging between $10,000 and
$13,000. As they do with other policies, both staffs democratically set their
own pay scale. By comparison, the fees and salaries of private practitioners and
government workers are much higher. Each Fort Helper who receivers a stipend is expected to match this from fees paid by those coming for help. About
twelve of the current (1980) staff receive no wages, including eight interns
from San Francisco State University and John F. Kennedy University.

About two-thirds of the staff are women, with most of the women and men
in their twenties and thirties although several are in the forties to seventies.
They come from predominantly white middle-class backgrounds. Despite the
flexibility and sacrifice still often required, only six people left the staff in 1979.
About three-fourths now have state licenses in various specialties, and others
are working towards masters degrees in psychology or marriage and family
counseling. Most have other part-time jobs and/or are going to school. Most
plan counseling careers; some are now doing part-time private practice, where
they usually reduce the fee for "clients" who are short of funds.

Some 150 persons with sex and relationship, suicide and depression, crime,
and other human problems; and 125 former heroin addicts on methadone
maintenance come to the center each week for low-cost, high-quality help.
The fees range from $8 to $35 ($45 for couples since it is based on joint income)
but even the $8 is sometimes waived when a person desperately needs help and
cannot afford to pay for it. The average fee seems to be $15. However, those on
the methadone program pay a flat $25 per week to cover the dispensing of
methadone in individualized doses, counseling, daily availability of staff, including weekends, and the weekly urine testing for drug use still required by
state and federal regulations. There is no fifty-minute hour but instead an emphasis on giving each individual, couple, or family the amount of time needed
from one or more staff members, one to several times each week. The guests

are predominantly white, but people continue to come in and be welcomed from a great diversity of cultural, racial, and religious backgrounds. They are mostly between the ages of nineteen and forty and mostly of lower socioeconomic status. But, of course, the boundaries of this have changed due to the on-going economic depression and growing unemployment. About thirty percent of those coming to the center for help are from the middle and sometimes upper classes.

In keeping with Joel's founding philosophy, there remains an emphasis on a person's strengths and on a humanistic, holistic, and eclectic helping approach. Long-term help is not stressed but is available. Special concern and availability of services remain for homosexuals and women along with men and heterosexuals. Various staff members are experienced with, and utilize, Gestalt, Jungian, nondirective, Reichian, psychosynthesis, Freudian, ego psychology, body work, and other techniques or approaches. There are fewer groups operating than at most times in the past, but the center counsels a steady number of couples, including some lesbian ones. There are special groups for overeaters (the obese), for women, and for men, but most people are helped on an individual basis. An unusual emphasis continues on connecting the person seeking help with the best person on the staff for the *guest*, with freedom of choice of counselor and type of help. Guests are able to ask for someone else if they are dissatisfied with some aspect of the help being provided them. Homosexuals are seen by either heterosexual or homosexual staff members, depending on the guest's preference. The courts are diverting some first time criminal offenders to Fort Help for rehabilitation.

There is a smooth relationship between the counseling and methadone maintenance subprograms. Most of the staff members dress informally, and none dresses or behaves in a manner that would separate them from other staff members or from the people coming to the center for help. More of the staff have a spouse and children than in the "old days." About five of the more experienced staff serve both as staff members and as consultants to other staff.

The singular openness about what we are doing continues with the weekly drop-in open house, where anyone from potential guests or staff to government agents can come anonymously and ask as many questions as they wish. Some visitors come at other times and from other parts of the country or other nations.

The large curved walls of the main living room have recently been painted with a beautiful mountain landscape by a San Francisco artist. The furnishings and decoration of the individual rooms remain simple and generally attractive, but the main floor needs carpeting badly, and the area of the center used by the methadone program remains drab. A plan to purchase the building in which the Fort is housed has been dropped because about three-fourths of the money which had been saved for that purpose was used for legal fees stemming from the false charges brought against us by the state health department and attorney general's office. For some there is an uncertainty about working here (will we have enough money? will we be able to stay here?). Up to this moment, however, we and our organizational philosophy have managed to cope with, and compensate for, the crises and the several major losses of income.

The governing or leadership of the center is done democratically by the staff, through weekly staff meetings which all are expected to attend and through committees or work groups called Assessment, Quality of Service, and Administration. The committees make recommendations to the larger staff, and a majority vote of those attending the staff meeting is needed for a policy change. For a time there were special committees for C.E.T.A. (Comprehensive Employment and Training Act, a government-sponsored program for training new workers) and for publicity. The publicity activities consisted of visiting other programs to explain Fort Help and its availability, arranging for some public service announcements on local radio and television stations, and putting small placards on San Francisco buses and trolleys. As in the past, people at the staff meetings question new ideas and talk at length, vote and re-vote, with everyone feeling responsibility for decisions. Many want to continue with what the center does well and are concerned that new programs or ventures may adversely affect that, but some respond quite positively to new ideas. Things sometimes don't get done unless by the person who initiates the proposal. Once a month the staff meeting involves a group encounter rather than a discussion of business. In order to be licensed as a community health clinic by the California Department of Health, the staff was required to name an "administrator" since all other organizations have one specific person that the health department can contact. R., a staff member doing both the accounting and counseling, accepted this role in name only for a year, but in practice functions no differently than other staff members and uses no regular title. A similar phenomenon exists in the methadone program, where state and federal regulations require all such program personnel to have fixed titles such as program director or medical director. So, qualified people accept such titles on paper, usually on a temporary or rotating basis, while in practice they continue democratic decision-making and equal pay for equal work.

The board of directors has met infrequently and irregularly in the last few years, but already has had two meetings in the first half of 1980. The board is moving in the direction of greater involvement in center activities; it added new members both from the community and the staff. Several members had resigned in response to the adversities experienced by the center, but active and constructive participation continues to be shown by such members as Owen Chamberlain, Arthur Lantz, Maria Fort, Karen Stone, Lothar Salin, and Joel Fort.

New people continue to apply by the dozens each year for staff membership and internships. Some are added gradually after careful assessment when current staff members leave (usually to make more money) or when a decision is made to have a greater number of people on the staff. New staff applicants are interviewed by three current staff members and are given direct feedback. About ten people have been accepted from those applying in recent months, and they have joined the staff. Quality is maintained by follow-up interviews at three months and one year by the assessment committee, which also receives reports and recommendations from the center's consultants. Staff work is also reevaluated and assessed at the time that they apply for a stipend. Additionally, each staff member is required to have an individual consultant and participate in a two-hour group each week to discuss cases and the treatment approaches being used. Periodic training to refine and develop skills is encouraged and provided at the center, or elsewhere at the center's expense. Staff members have occasional parties. After a long absence of this particular practice, the staff went on a weekend retreat in June, 1980.

During the year prior to completion of this book the staff did a number of special things, including the community outreach effort already mentioned, an art therapy exercise focusing on individual visions of the Fort's future, a program on play therapy, a movie series for the community, support groups for diabetics, relaxation exercises, and the continued defense against the Medi-Cal charges. There is talk of doing more training, of trying to get more recognition for the many valuable achievements, opening an annex, soundproofing the rooms, and helping more guests, including more middle-income people, as government services are cut back and/or as more "casualties" from private practitioners come in.

The methadone maintenance program, originally named the Antiaddiction and Methadone Maintenance Program, is still the only nongovernmental, nonprofit program in the state, and like the rest of Fort Help it remains the only democratically operated one in the country. Unlike the rest of the center, much of what the methadone program does is controlled by rigid state and national laws and regulations, with an accompanying network of overlapping enforcers. The regulations have remained essentially unchanged since 1973, including the requirement of weekly urine testing for opiates, barbiturates, amphetamines, and methadone. This regulation remains despite a 1978 study of the effectiveness of urine monitoring done by the state at five participating clinics including Fort Help. Control subjects continued to provide urine samples while experimental subjects had no urine testing during the one-year study. Both groups showed about the same percentage of illicit drug use, thus proving that urine testing is unnecessary (as well as expensive and degrading), as Joel had long claimed.

Two staff members serve on the Task Force for the California Department of Alcohol and Drug Programs, and several former staff members now lead other methadone programs in the state. Of the some 125 people on the program, most are white, but there are ten chicanos and five blacks; about sixty percent are male; and most live in San Francisco, although some come from the East Bay and from Marin County to the north. All but fifty receive some take-home doses of methadone (which requires consistently "clean" urines), so they need not come in every day for the drug. They find the place nicer and more accessible, less threatening, and unbureaucratic compared to other programs. Only thirty are unemployed. About two-thirds have been in continuous treatment for less than two years, with the dose of methadone usually ranging between sixty and one hundred milligrams daily.

This extensive and complex, private nonprofit organization continues to operate at low cost (See Appendix I). In 1979, the general helping program of the center (not including methadone maintenance) had total revenues of $95,783.43, of which nearly $87,000 came from fees. The expenses during the same period were $112,760.12, with the three major items being more than $62,000 for staff stipends, $14,000 for rent and $13,000 in legal fees. The net deficit for the year was taken care of through the modest reserves from previous years, still leaving a small reserve of $5,751.63.

Other things happen, including many career transformations. One person, for example, went from being a receptionist at an ultra-traditional university mental health program to a current counseling and leadership position at the Fort with a masters degree and licensing in marriage and family counseling. Telephone help remains extensive, and there are still no secretaries. Smoking is still prohibited.

No media attention has been directed to the many positive and unique achievements of the center, its staff, or its founder. In part, this is because the present staff has not solicited the media as do other organizations, private and public. Also, in part, there is a negative perception of the media for having singled out and attacked the center in conjunction with the Medi-Cal fiasco.

As for the program ancestors of Fort Help created by Joel, the Mobile Help Unit ended when the San Francisco poverty program changed administrators and turned it into a regular vehicle for transporting people. The National Sex and Drug Forum became simply the National Sex Forum. It continues training people to work in the sex field, but in a more formal way with credit courses and diplomas. Most of the medical school and other college sexuality courses, now common in America, stem from the National Sex Forum, along with a large library of sex education films distributed through the now-separate Multi-Media Center. The series of all day encounter workshops in San Francisco and New York between police and revolutionaries (and once between a sheriff and his deputies) were not continued. It culminated in a one hour television documentary and a half hour film, "To Make a Start in Ending Violence," which is circulated by Psychological Films.

The most direct antecedent of Fort Help is the original San Francisco Health Department's Center for Special Problems. It originated in 1965 and has now survived almost fifteen years. Analagous (except financially) to an occasional playwright, Joel has two "hit" programs running simultaneously.

The Center for Special Problems serves more than two thousand different people yearly in providing psychological and medical services, including drug treatment, as a speciality mental health clinic of the city. It continues to deal with problems of sex, gender, drugs, and crime. The annual report states that it has "assumed the primary coordinating role in developing mental health services for San Francisco gay residents" (a logical consequence of being in 1965 the first public clinic for homosexuals and transsexuals). The health department's center utilizes Fort Help as a primary referral place for victims of sexual assault or other violent crimes, as well as for detoxification of drug abusers and hormones for transsexuals. The city-county program has a community advisory board, a staff, training program, and placement for graduate students. The annual budget has grown to about $735,000, of which $400,000 is reimbursed by Medi-Cal collections. However, because of tax cuts, there was a reduction of $125,000, including six positions, in 1980. Also, this center has been shifted administratively to a new forensic mental health section in the department of public health, and will be accepting only the emotionally disturbed person who is involved in the criminal justice system. A social worker hired there by Joel as the first acknowledged (by him and the city) homosexual in the civil service system has become director in recent years, also thus showing that non-physicians are qualified for these administrative positions.

Chapter 6
SPECIAL LEARNINGS

The deepest problems of modern life derive from the claim of the individual to preserve the autonomy and individuality of existence in the face of overwhelming social forces. —Simmel

The development of a new social organization requires as much creativity and perseverance as the creation of a symphony or painting, we believe. It is really social artistry. There is also the parallel of loneliness and sacrifice experienced by writers, artists, and composers, whether with a masterpiece or a failure. Unless one is a self-publicist, there is little recognition to be expected in nontraditional approaches, or ones that go against the powerful institutions and illusions of society. At the least this includes organized medicine and psychiatry, the drug and sex police, some political extremists, and many government health administrators.

Fort Help wanted to help people of all backgrounds and ages cope better with the many problems of living, and to enhance their potential. Mental, emotional, and behavioral problems were, to the early coleaders of the center, not the symptoms of vague and stigmatizing mental illness but rather the self-defeating results of social learning in a dehumanizing environment. Thus, back in the 1960s, a humanistic, holistic and radical (attacking the root causes) center was brought into being. Illness, treatments, and treaters were demystified and demythologized, and emphasis was shifted to the social causes and to people's ability and responsibility to help themselves. As in the medical speciality of public health, the focus was on prevention and on immunizing people against pathological social forces. It turned out to be the right program and philosophy

61

but, in our judgment, in the wrong time and, perhaps, the wrong city. The fault may lie not in the stars but in the developers, for ignoring the politics of success and the necessary liaisons with media and others of the power structure.

No matter how lofty its ideals and purpose, an organization needs to maintain contact with, and extract energy from, the world surrounding it if it is to survive. This includes being able to solve problems of finances and public image. Unless sufficient funds are generated to keep the operation afloat, it will founder; unless people are aware of the organization's existence in a positive way, it is unlikely they will come to it or otherwise support it.

From the very beginning, we chose a path that brought with it independence and financial uncertainty. Joel's past experience with government funding had convinced him that such funds are not only capriciously awarded and undependable for continuation, but that the controlling strings attached to them make it virtually impossible to do the creative and democratic things that we felt ethics and professional standards require. The government expects the "piper to be paid" handsomely. If one accepts its money one generally winds up doing what it wants, no matter how far removed that may be from what one had in mind to begin with or what is ideal for the people one is committed to serve.

We have a further strong conviction that good programs need to be based on a knowledgeable and dedicated staff. It is *people* who come first—money, buildings, equipment, and highly paid administrators are a distant second or third. A good program will attract and hold people at financial compensation levels far lower than what conventional operations have to offer. Those whose sense of worth is based solely on money are often merely time servers anyway, and we need to counteract the trends of a society which is overly mercantile, is oriented towards hucksterism, and is quantity-bigness-money-obsessed. In the San Francisco city-county government program he had created in 1965, out of a moribund traditional clinic, Joel had tripled the case load and increased tenfold the kinds of problems served, the hours open, the number of staff, and the outreach services, without any increase in budget. Yet, many of the ideas, innovations, experiments, and iconoclasms that have become part and parcel of Fort Help were things that the top city-county health administrators had rejected in 1967 after they were tried or proposed at the Center for Special Problems.

The Fort Help experience has been that an outstanding program can attract people of the highest caliber without offering large financial rewards, but that it is not possible to hold them indefinitely without some sort of adequate compensation. In the absence of a policy that at least begins to meet financial needs as well as intellectual and emotional ones, the people who will remain the longest are only occasionally the most capable ones. It is both a matter of altruism and dedication and of available choices.

If government agencies and mental health facilities were offering services mandated by the taxpayers' support and delivering services that high professional and ethical standards require, there would be little need or place for new and alternative agencies. Thus, the answer to the "why" of Fort Help starts with services being nonexistent or inadequate. It began in the 1960s, survived and flourished through the 1970s, and continues now into the 1980s—bloodied, different, and helping. No public program or private psychiatrists, psychologists, or social workers, including the precursor Center for Special Problems, were responding adequately to the large and rapidly growing problems of drug abuse, sexuality, obesity, suicide, and violence. None was dealing with these concerns in an integrated, comprehensive way. None was operating in a nonauthoritarian way and few in a nonpsychiatric way. None existed without accumulating and/or spending large amounts of money. None gave people of all backgrounds an opportunity for leadership and creative social involvement.

There were many positive rewards and personal as well as organizational satisfactions at Fort Help, and luckily these far outweighed the absence of financial rewards. Countless people formed friendships that still endure years after their association here. Even more received experience (or training) that made their future careers possible.

The best part of the whole range of social contacts was that most of the time there were interesting, alert, creative people on staff with whom it was easy to want to be friends. Perhaps it was because we were all there voluntarily and with a shared sense of community. (There were also a few who were difficult to get along with, but we believe that you don't need to like someone to cooperate with them for a broader purpose.)

The simple fact of establishing Fort Help and keeping it operating for ten years, enabling an extremely heterogeneous staff to perform services for which degrees and licenses are required elsewhere, is an achievement in itself. The many thousands of guests seen (and more talked to on the phone) more cost effectively than by traditional clinics justify our efforts to insure the survival of the center during its early days and years. In addition, the work at Fort Help enabled some twenty of us to eventually acquire those degrees and licenses in order to do the same kind of work elsewhere.

The functioning of the organization as a help center, however, as important as it is and was, is less significant to society in the long run than the lessons to be learned from its organization and structure.

SOME ACCOMPLISHMENTS

Joel once wrote for a staff meeting the following list of major accomplishments of the Center for Solving Problems—Fort Help:

1. Provided help and hope to many thousands of people, face-to-face and by phone, with a great diversity of problems, backgrounds, and ages.

2. Served a wide range of human problems: sex, relationship, drugs, suicide, pregnancy, obesity, crime, etc., in one place without becoming isolated.

3. Survived for more than six years (at time of the meeting) of a very ambitious, complex, and comprehensive program and without accepting government funding and control or using public relations or the media—all in marked contrast to other programs.

4. Proved that a nonhierarchical, nonbureaucratic organization can work and be as efficient as a conventional bureaucracy while proving much less expensive and more fun.

5. Accomplished a unique and successful blending of staff with and without degrees, paid and unpaid, of ages eighteen to seventy, in a new concept of volunteerism and professionalism without professional or bureaucratic titles, with flexi-scheduling, and with one's sense of worth coming from doing something relevant and altruistic rather than from money.

6. Provided equality and leadership for women and men, the young and older.

7. Provided equality and leadership for homosexuals and heterosexuals, male and female.

8. Proved that a nonmedical, nonpsychiatric, nonsickness model of helping works and is well-accepted—perhaps the first actual humanistic clinic.

9. Provided a smorgasbord, eclectic helping-approach encouraging drop-ins, freedom of choice, informality, accessibility.

10. Gave an opportunity to staff for growth, training including apprenticeships, new careers, friendships, and sometimes love.

11. Trained hundreds who have gone on to other programs and careers, and in general demonstrated new approaches which, in part, have been taken up by many agencies and individuals in the United States and abroad.

12. Made unusual use of the physical environment to humanize and informalize help—"living rooms," individually decorated smaller private rooms with names, color, etc.

13. Gave extensive telephone help, both crisis and long-term counseling.

14. Expressed concern about quality of services and staff, with high ethical standards including no sexual exploitation of guests, no violence, and no smoking at the center.

We could easily conclude our review and summary at this point and say: "It couldn't be done—but it was; a staff of fifty or sixty people cannot function without tight administration—but they did; a nontraditional, nonprofessional place can't last—but it did!" Quantitatively, the dream has been achieved many times over, and since hardly anyone besides Joel *really* expected this to happen, we could leave it at that. Many staff members have never considered it possible or even desirable to strive for more or even as much. There is, however, the ideal Joel refers to in his visionary statement of 1970, as "a place where we *pursue excellence* and seek mutual tolerance of different life-styles." From a *qualitative* point of view, these goals had a checkered history of achievement.

LEADERSHIP, ORGANIZATION, AND INDIVIDUAL LEARNINGS

The heart of the Fort Help experience was the day-to-day work and the way in which we organized ourselves and shared the leadership to perform our work (see Appendix J). The first thing that comes to mind to describe this experience is the term *alternative*, but it was much more than that. Almost everyone on the staff stresses the fact that what made Fort Help interesting, different, and effective was its nonbureaucratic, humanistic, and democratic nature.

There is sharing of work, lack of administrative structure, taking care of staff social needs, dealing with many of people's problems, providing a place for talented nonlicensed people to work, group decision-making—all these frequently competing and conflicting ideals and practices were what individual staff people were looking for. A democratic method of organization has its limitations in a work context, but the usual authoritarian organization has even more limitations, and is less fun.

WORK STRUCTURE

The staff leadership should never have abolished the "indirect services" category of staff and permitted only direct services by greeter-problem-solvers. There is no way an individual, without some years of training and/or experience, can be an effective generalist (counselor, therapist), greeter (intake worker, crisis intervention helper), telephone helper and coleader of a complex organization all at the same time. Trying to force this assures mediocre performance at some levels, especially when people are expected to work for low or no pay. Too much homogenization prevents some people from becoming either outstanding generalists, superb greeters, or inspirational leaders. Paradoxically, the opportunity and encouragement to do so produced some outstanding all-around women and men.

As to moderate or low stipends, Joel prefers to talk of "professional work without large salaries or titles." The difference is more than just semantic. Lothar considered anything significantly less than what one commands under conventional circumstances (for instance, $10 hourly compensation for someone who can easily earn two or three times that) to be "volunteer work." A problem arises when other staff members, for whom $4 or $5 an hour may be top pay, consider this "a large salary."

It is interesting to note that as much as we deemphasized professional degrees per se, almost two-thirds of the longtime key staff members ended up acquiring degrees and/or licences during or since their association with the center. Also, more than a third of the staff, in addition to their counseling, participated in real leadership roles—a phenomenal percentage—and the rest participated to a limited extent.

The original goals were, of course, Joel's, but after the initial years, they became ours. He largely declined participation in formal and lengthy discussions, along with more than half of the continuing staff who left meetings to others, preferring to go about their work instead. Occasional mass meetings, including partially recreational retreats, both set and attempted to implement goals. We believe that the people who carry out the work must be involved in the setting of the goals at the start.

Lothar proposed an analysis based on management theory: alternative/futuristic organizations can occur with two very different goals in mind, namely, the performance of services or good feelings among the staff. The latter goal is the result of what can be called *country-club management*, and fails for the same reason. If people not only set their own goals but also evaluate and generally make things as easy as possible on themselves, in the mistaken notion that this will make them more productive, it will largely induce them to do as little as they can get away with. The pitfall to be avoided is, of course, McGregor's Theory X, the restrictive, coercive, hard-driving "bossism" style of management. Its opposite is *not* total permissiveness but Theory Y, which presumes positive as well as negative motivation factors among workers and provides reinforcement for the former. There can be a Theory Y in an alternative setting, but like its counterpart in traditional settings it has to be carefully worked out with planning and, above all, the presence of more than one entity of decision-making power.

BOARD OF DIRECTORS

Some boards err in becoming personally involved in the day-to-day running of the program. But this was never our problem. Very few members of our board of directors performed actual services for us, and a bare quorum showed up for the board meetings three times a year. The board could have been set up differently in order to make it function more actively and to provide stability for the staff. One possibility would have been to create a separate advisory board and a working board. The latter would include both outsiders with decision-making expertise who are willing to come to regular monthly meetings, and a limited number of present or former staff. Such a working board could act more effectively, not just in monitoring overall policies but also in taking care of things which the staff as a whole had little or no interest in or aptitude for, such as large-scale fund-raising and relations with the media.

PUBLIC EDUCATION

Providing general information, or public education, our major means of contact with the outer world apart from our guests and staff, was intermittent and minimal except for Joel's frequent lecturing, locally and nationally, up to 1975. For about the first year of our operation, we were fortunate to have a professional copywriter on staff in the person of T., who went on to study counseling and is now in private practice. T. typed and mimeographed everything that was needed, with input from Joel, Meg, and Lothar. The regular appearance of newsletters during the early days was an important part of our internal communication and openness with each other.

For external purposes, a brochure describing our services and philosophy was put together: first a rudimentary one in black and white, then a two-color version. During early 1971, we had a stroke of luck in that the San Francisco Junior Advertising Club (advertising people under age thirty) adopted Fort Help as its yearly part-time project. The project involved the creation of a complete multimedia campaign of ads, billboard designs, cards for public transportation vehicles, a distinctive Fort Help logo, stationery, and radio public service announcements. Unfortunately, we were largely a vehicle for the advertising club to develop a model campaign which it could enter in a national competition among all junior ad clubs. The emphasis, therefore, was on what looked and sounded good, not on what was practical. We received a good logo and slogan, "*Help Without Hassle*," as well as finished ad layouts and professionally-recorded, creative radio spots. What we did *not* receive were the applications: we got billboard layouts that could be translated into actual billboards if we wanted and could pay for them, show-cards that we could not afford to print and display in buses, and so on. The whole campaign provided us with a boost in morale, but the major tangible result was a first prize for the ad club in the national contest. In our entire history, this was the only thing approaching formal public relations.

Not surprisingly, the most noticeable channel of public or community relations has been by word of mouth. Over the years, many thousands have used Fort Help's drop-in and telephone-advice services since we serve anybody, anywhere. In addition, several thousand come by appointment for on-going help. Guests have come from all over the Bay Area and, sometimes, from other parts of California and the United States. Also, we have had many professional visitors from France, Japan, Australia, and other countries. The comments of guests and visitors have not only reached friends and acquaintances but, along with staff contacts, have had some impact on those who work at other community facilities, in private practice, or teach and supervise in institutions of higher learning.

In the beginning, of course, we had no public reputation at all, and the very idea of a nonbureaucratic, nongovernmental, health and growth-oriented center that went beyond degrees and licenses was viewed with considerable skepticism by the professional community. It took most of two years to establish the fact that Fort Help was indeed a place where serious work was done, much of it of a high quality. The center is presently well-regarded and used for self-referrals and referrals by many other agencies. Despite a lack of media support, and some attacks, Fort Help has carved a niche for itself. We think that represents a solid achievement.

STAFF PROFILE

It is difficult to say what kind of a staff profile, long-term or short-term, emerges. The original staff was a heterogeneous and creative mix of people, sometimes short on skills but long on enthusiasm. There were also highly-trained professionals, tired of stifling atmospheres and eager to do something new. As we progressed and needed more people who could do serious work well, we accepted more people with experience from the relatively large numbers who continued to apply, and apprenticed some who were not yet fully qualified.

Slowly, starting in 1972, a new staff philosophy emerged which was, at first, laughingly regarded as "the poverty ethic." Many kinds of people staffed the Fort: comfortable middle class, poor, hip, activists, experienced therapist-counselors, apprentices, middle-aged, young. Life-style had always been a matter of personal choice; our concern has been with the quality of the work, not with any irrelevant idiosyncrasies of sex, color, age, or degrees. The newer ethic was that one had to actively deprive oneself to be a "real Fort Helper." Although significant altruism and sacrifice were already present in most staff members, this ethic slowly gained acceptance and was one of the several factors that changed the composition of the staff. We weathered the resulting dissension, as we had other troubles. Some of the less experienced staff went back to school, and a large number of graduate students chose Fort Help as their field placement for new and serious work.

Those who found satisfaction, by and large, were self-starters. Structure at Fort Help stressed individual responsibility and accountability, initiative, and ability. People with a "take care of me" attitude were largely disappointed. A successful staffer in need of training would take the initiative and arrange for the kind of help he or she wanted.

A few words should be said about the concept of experience. This does not mean degrees and licenses. The Assessment Committee turned down several applicants with master's and doctoral credentials who appeared too rigid or traditional to fit our requirements. Nor does experience mean simply having been around. Someone may have worked at free or mental health clinics or in private practice for several years, and therefore be experienced, but this does not necessarily mean that he or she is *good* and ethical at work. Experience does imply, however, the achievement of a goal, a certain amount of discipline in attaining this goal, and some self-imposed but recognizable standards. We began to have problems when we accepted people who "talked good jargon" but otherwise failed to meet other standards.

Our insistence on new staff with experience was based on the realization that we simply did not have the time and energy needed to do constant in-depth training for total beginners. For one reason or another, there was always attrition; every time we thought we had a good overall staff, one or two key people would leave. They had found a paying job; their involvement at school or with other things had become too great; or, rarely, they got tired of us. Sometimes the turnover slowed, and several months would go by with only one or two people leaving. But we were obliged to maintain a constant process of staff replenishment. While we tried to hire those who could go right to work unsupervised, we always tried to meet the needs of someone who, once on staff, turned out to be less capable than we thought, as long as he or she wanted to learn.

CREATIVITY

In 1976, Joel raised the question of whether the many talented people who left Fort Help did so because they outgrew it (as they usually put it) or because they sought more income, security, and status (as he suggested). The major satisfactions connected with Fort Help were helping a wide variety of people, controlling one's own destiny, doing innovative work, and creating a utopian system. To these eventually was added the possibility of accruing valuable hours of experience towards one's private practice license. To some people, this would not seem enough reward for a lot of hard work. It is almost surprising, therefore, that so many people stayed for such a long time; but it is also not surprising that many left, even though their continued presence was still important.

Lothar believes that truly creative people are not only used to, but *entitled* to, a certain amount of preferential treatment since their contribution to the totality of the effort is great but often intangible. Refusing them this tangible *quid pro quo* amounts to exploitation of the talented by the needy. If the creative person has any choice, he or she will leave. This process ultimately results in the group's losing the services of the talented person altogether. The second law of thermodynamics, which prescribes that the nature of systems is to settle into quiet and uniformity, is reinforced by eliminating the antientropic stimuli which is provided by the creative person.

BOOKKEEPING

One of the areas in which there has been a steady improvement over the years has been financial efficiency and responsibility. In the early days, bookkeeping was sporadic and mostly nonexistent. We had little money or income; there were always bills to pay. The coordinators paid what they could whenever they got around to it, and hoped for the best. The financial mess of the methadone program in 1971 was partly due to the fact that no one was closely supervising how much money should have been collected, how much actually came in, and how much we could afford to spend. A potentially useful idea suggested by Joel and implemented by Meg and him, the use of Mastercharge and BankAmerica cards by guests, never found much acceptance by the staff.

Following the financial crisis of 1971, and the resulting reorganization, we instituted careful accounting and bookkeeping procedures. H. was originally paid out of methadone funds to keep track of that program's income and disbursements, and she eventually did the accounts for all of Fort Help. The system for this had been set up long before by one of our early staff, S., a very capable accountant who donated his professional expertise and supervision. Unfortunately, the complex demands of Fort Help's finances went far beyond the abilities of the then mostly unpaid staff, who tried to do it on a part-time basis knowing little of accounting principles. In the summer of 1973, J., an unemployed school teacher, was hired to do the bookkeeping for a period.

In 1974, R. signed on as bookkeeper when J. decided to become an apprentice counselor instead. Since R. combines a communal lifestyle in yoga and an accounting degree, this turned out to be a happy choice. For the first time, financial statements (quarterly at first, monthly before too long) became a regular Fort Help procedure. We learned the difference between cash and accruals and how to budget for recurrent items. In the long run, the pragmatic needs for financial accountability overcame the reluctance to create even one part-time specialized position. However, the bookkeepers became other things as well, including valued counselor helpers.

SERVICE DOCUMENTATION

Recordkeeping and statistics, by design, have never been a major part of the Fort Help scene, but several detailed documents (evaluations) exist. The first was an in-depth longitudinal study of Lothar's cases, made as part of his master's thesis in 1973. Another, largely compiled by J. and the Quality of Service group in 1975, quantifies as much as possible the available data on new guests coming to the center during a two-month period (see Appendix K). As J. indicated, during many months there were more than one hundred new greetings, in addition to the hundreds coming weekly for on-going services. After early 1975, the percentage of substantially employed guests able to pay appropriate fees increased greatly.

SUPPORT AND MAINTENANCE TASKS

One of the principal illusions of the nonbureaucratic, alternative model of organization is the expectation that somehow everyone will recognize the tasks that need covering, without one person being made responsible for them. The reality is that there are certain tasks that are too boring, too demanding, or too specialized to have much appeal. Included are secretarial or clerical tasks, as well as housekeeping and cleaning. Sometimes staff members just stepped around trash, and ignored the cigarette butts. Then we would hold a meeting at which we agreed that "everyone needed to take more responsibility." At another time, we decided that some nonpaying clients could barter for their services by doing cleanup work. When this didn't produce enough results, those who needed money were allowed to divide the work among themselves. Eventually we decided to establish a janitorial contract (briefly with an outside firm, then with two people on staff) for specific services and standards. Then the place was kept clean.

Most people confuse effectiveness and efficiency. Fort Help attacked the latter, mainly emphasizing humane effectiveness in helping people to solve a wide range of human problems. Using both men and women in clerical positions would be another way of eliminating sexism. However, everybody, regardless of position, needs to be able to do their own basic clerical and support work. There is no reason not to dial most of one's own telephone calls, type some letters, or make one's own coffee. Equally important, this independence brings a sharp drop in paperwork and the time-consuming minutiae of organizational life. When it becomes a matter of tracking someone down by telephone at several locations or preparing a lengthy document for presentation, on the other hand, we may waste valuable decision-making or counseling time on routine tasks.

PHILOSOPHY

In order to understand the functioning of an organization, one has to come to grips with its philosophy in addition to its staff, services and procedures. This is one of the areas in which Fort Help is well-documented. The goals are numerous, although sometimes difficult to put into practice. People of very divergent personal belief structures appropriated that part of the philosophy to which they related and followed it as *the* Fort Help way, conveniently forgetting other parts that were unrelated or in conflict with their beliefs.

Joel has a personal, dedicated crusade against smoking, but the rest of his ethics appeal strongly to people who are nicotine addicts. Thus, it took almost three years to keep all staff and guests from smoking on the premises, in spite of the fact that this had been an avowed part of our philosophy from the very beginning. We lost some talented people this way, as we did from our emphasis on equality for women, nonprofessionalism, and homosexuals. Some were bitter at being "forced" off the staff over what they considered a "petty" issue.

Another example of how a broad general philosophy can wind up embracing several competing tunnel-visions concerns political orientation. Joel is not just a generalist but a synthesizer, sometimes seeming to straddle what is to some an ideological Grand Canyon. One of our major problems seemed to come from failing to understand that when Joel attacked the dehumanizing aspects of modern mass society, it was a roundhouse swing at *all* existing closed, sterile systems and particularly all totalitarianism. It called for something totally new. What we were trying to do at Fort Help was very different from the standard approach of "radical therapy" or "conservative therapy." We did not believe in superimposing a particular, limited set of political or psychiatric values on the helping situation. Joel has never used words like liberal, left-wing, right-wing, conservative, Freudian, Marxist, or collective—preferring specificity and individualism that goes beyond ideology and polarization.

Few of us recognized sufficiently that among the noisy radical fringe surrounding us, constantly harping about power trips and authoritarianism, were also well-disciplined collectivists and totalitarians to whom our democratic concepts meant dangerous individual choice and freedom. We intermittently saw a few examples on our staff. The kind of help we tried to give is simply not separable from an overall philosophy of living.

We operated on the basis that the ultimate resource resides in the individual, the personal responsibility of the man or woman we were trying to help. Otherwise, those aspects become emphasized that make the guest a victim and urge him or her to seek salvation by adjustment to a benevolent group or ideology (psychological, religious, or political). While there are many operational theories, any operational structure can be evaluated appropriately only in the ultimate crucible of *results*. No amount of free-flowing style, desirability, recognition of human values, opening of communication channels, or even sound practices, will stand very long in the absence of outstanding results.

SERVICES VERSUS MANAGEMENT

Any organization that exists to provide services cannot afford the luxury, and does not have the right, to be evaluated primarily in terms of how growth-producing a process it is for staff. More importantly, the principal rationale for an alternative organization to begin with is that it will lead to *improved services*. Administrative structure, which is, after all, only the secondary underpinning of the rendering of services, should be minimal but it cannot be nonexistent. At the point where one notices that things are not functioning well, it is necessary to start modifying the original model. It is essential for the creation of a service-oriented structure not to make the mistake of confusing divergency of skills on a functional level with administrative hierarchy. As a minimum, the division of duties should include two direct service categories (greeter/problem-solver and therapist/counselor/generalist), an indirect services category, and apprentices to all. One can function well without highly paid administrators.

The traditional corporate and governmental setting—one based on exaggerating inequalitites and politics rather than on talent—has a "slave system" much less effective and pleasant than our approach. But all are not created equal; there are indeed inequalitites of talent, performance, and creativity that need to be functionally reflected in the structure. Neither inhumanity nor mediocrity should be acceptable.

Excellence and egalitarianism can turn out to be poorly compatible. To excel means to stand out, which is hard to do in an atmosphere where one concept of egalitarianism is pushed. Also, the more effort that needs to be expanded in fighting this conflict, the less energy and inclination remain to do those things one can excel at.

REFLECTIONS

Besides the frustration over the nonrealization of some goals and the failure to achieve all-around excellence, we raise the point whether, after ten years or more, significantly innovative work is still likely to happen unless the organization is regenerated by new staff. Some of the formerly advanced thinking at Fort Help has now become broadly accepted. We have witnessed the undue publicity about whether someone, following a sex change operation, can be allowed to participate in women's tennis tournaments. Homosexuals have now been voted into a nonsickness diagnostic category by the American Psychiatric Association. The medical model in the mental health field, too, has been softened and modified by less judgmental, less rigid, interdisciplinary approaches.

Marxism, an oft-proposed solution to perennial problems, basically revives the medieval (class system) organization of humans in its most oppressive aspects without any redeeming qualities. It not only decries individual achievement but is basically born of despair. While Marxism or fascism may wind up being the only option in a grossly overpopulated and underdeveloped society, it represents a sad step backwards for those who have known and enjoyed extensive freedom and technology. To present totalitarianism as an innovative alternative is a fraud, particularly when one realizes the extreme bureaucratic nature of such societies.

We need other successful models of alternative organization like Fort Help in order to channel the frustrations and energies of modern society beyond the tyrannies of both the corporate and the collective world. The desire to achieve, to experience one's talents at full strength, while trying to do the "impossible" is what has made our evolution from the apes possible. The capable individual and program make a difference, but the bureaucratic and political world blocks and transforms capability and idealism. This age-old struggle may well continue as long as there are human beings, but Fort Help represents the wave of the future. It may make these recurrent polarized struggles obsolete. It can foster high creativity and altruism without the unhealthy side-effects of traditional organizations.

Santayana, as well as Nietzsche, has pointed out that people are condemned to act out the same mistakes again and again through their ignorance of history (and their destructiveness). "The miracle on Eleventh Street," as Joel once called it, can make others' efforts at building new private and public organizations much easier. Gandhi was once asked by a reporter what he thought of western civilization. His response was, "It would be nice."

Tolstoy told us that the only basic questions for humans are how to live and what to live for. But an important component of that is the way people organize themselves to work. Bennis, writing in 1964 and 1970 about a post-bureaucratic society, first foresaw new organizations with human and democratic ideals rather than depersonalized mechanistic bureacracies; but he then realized this had not occurred and that we had not substituted collaboration and reason for coercion and fear. Both Fromm and Argyris have raised doubts about the psychological attractiveness of democracy in organizations. Democracy does not seem "sexy" enough and is unable to engender the deep emotional commitments and satisfactions that authoritarian ideological movements do. The discontinuity between micro and macro systems, and the preponderance of individual greed over public interest, greatly hinder reforms, let alone revolutions in bureaucracy. Michael, another respected theorist of bureaucracy, calls for long-term education to bring about empathy, compassion, trust, nonexploitation, nonmanipulation, self-growth, tolerance for ambiguity, acknowledgement of error, and patience in employees and their organizations.

Toffler, in popularizing the concept of future shock, talks of moving beyond bureaucracy to adaptive, rapidly changing temporary systems where problems are solved by task forces of relative strangers representing diverse professional skills. He cites Weber's predicting the ultimate triumph of classical bureaucracy, and more recent figures predicting its demise in twenty-five years not because of humanistic or Christian values, but because of its inability to adapt to rapid change. Instead of organization men or women oriented to their own security through subordinating themselves, he thinks there will be an "adhocracy" with reduced group cohesiveness and commitment to work groups, a rise in professional rather than organizational loyalty, a move beyond narrow disciplines, a new venturesome spirit rather than security-minded conformity/orthodoxy, and self-motivated, coequal associates rather than vertically organized subordinates.

Slater proposes that the worth of organizations should be evaluated by how much pleasure or satisfaction they have given to people. Forrester suggests that organizations will eventually eliminate the superior-subordinate relationship and substitute individual self-discipline arising from self-interest. Argyris, writing prolifically since the mid-1960s about "tomorrow's organizations," predicted a revolution in the introduction of new organizations replacing the traditional ones in order for business organizations to survive in an increasingly competitive environment, and because of the newly available information technology. A traditional bureaucratic structure causes constant interdepartmental, win-lose competition while depending on conformity, mistrust, and selfishness. He thinks that the matrix organization, which started with large government defense projects, is a promising strategy to induce integration and cooperation in business organizations. This involves project teams created to solve particular problems, using people representing all relevant managerial functions. Each member is given equal responsibility and power to solve the problem, while being expected to work cohesively—and then disband, moving on to new assignments when the problem is solved. An organization may have a number of such teams, each led by a project manager. Taken together they constitute what is called a matrix.

In studying nine large organizations, Argyris found it difficult for them to put these concepts into practice due to people still polarizing issues, resisting new ideas, mistrusting others, protecting their own survival, oversimplifying criteria of success, focusing on the short-term and the team, worrying about recognition, bogging down on what had not been accomplished — in other words, the negative. He concludes that changing the organization greatly increases the tension level; so in order to counter restraining forces, the basic values of executives have to be altered over and beyond changing the structure of the organization. Different leadership styles seem to him to be needed by different organizations: authoritarian for traditional bureaucracies; participative for linchpin organizations proposed by Likert; and risk-taking, trusting leadership for matrix organizations.

The executive of the future will learn to develop an organizational environment that challenges people, stretches their aspirations, and develops a productive tension which an individual can control and use to increase his or her competencies. Up to half the meetings and three-quarters of the time spent in meetings are unproductive and unnecessary, in today's organizations. Major organizational reformers have difficulty foreseeing all the problems involved, the extraordinary amount of time needed to work out the obstacles and gain acceptance of the changes, and the lack of commitment of many people to make a new plan work. With thirty-two organizations where he had consulted, Argyris did not find one reorganization completed and integrated after three years.

Sale, in the most recent major book that is pertinent to making dreams reality, describes a "beanstalk principle"—when governments become centralized and enlarged beyond a limited range, they not only stop solving problems but begin to create them. There is an optimal limit beyond which organizations should not grow. He finds all bureaucracies to have considerable deficiencies, with the govenment ones, the largest, having the most due to civil-service protection, large tax-supported budgets, and weak legislative review. They are characteristically inflexible, uncreative, unproductive, self-protective, inefficient, irresponsible, and authoritarian. During their hours of employment, such employees forego most of the democratic values we purport to believe in: free speech, free assembly, free press, privacy, and due process. They are not represented in the financial or decision-making processes, cannot challenge decisions made by a handful of distant people whom they did not elect and cannot remove, and function at the whim of superiors. Other authorities, too, highlight the theme that we have repeatedly stressed—that bureaucracy is the enemy of individual liberty, transferring control from the people to a class of professional technicians, who, as Nisbet puts it, substitute their organizations, their tastes, and their aspirations for ours.

These situations continue, despite the findings of national polls that suggest large majorities of people in America prefer individual expression to group experience, want to participate in community decisions, like cooperation better than competition, welcome challenges, think that technology has caused as many problems as benefits, think it is more important to learn to live with basics rather than achieve higher living standards, prefer human over material values, and are ready to change their life-style.

Chapter 7
IMPLICATIONS FOR NEW DREAMERS

The hottest places in hell are reserved for those who in times of great moral crisis do nothing. —Dante

Out of all this, some very specific implications emerge for other organizations that would like to use the Fort Help model—operate with creative principles and avoid an administrative hierarchy—yet be even better staffed, trained, and supervised. Even so, we did more than enough to gain what we regard as a national reputation for significant and excellent work. For whatever the value, we serve as a model for creating and revitalizing organizations.

GOALS

Most of our goals have been and are now implicitly part of the operational philosophy of the center. Here is a formalization of our credo:

1. Use a nonjudgmental approach as the basis of the helping process, rejecting medical/psychiatric models or techniques, personality theories, or length of helping relationships.

2. Work with as little structure as possible, largely sharing administrative work and decision-making powers, without, however, rejecting functional organization where it serves a necessary purpose.

3. Firmly reject, without exception, sexual involvement between staff and guests.

4. No smoking on or near the premises.

5. Be open with each other and concentrate on honest personal interaction among staff, without letting this take precedence over services to guests.

6. Respect all life-styles, personal values, social or political views, and sexual orientations; do not discriminate against any group as a class.

7. Do not be satisfied with mere adequacy, but strive at all times for the outstanding.

8. While believing in a multiplicity of possible personal value systems within this framework and encouraging experimentation with new ideas, nevertheless recognize that these listed values and goals are non-negotiable and those who cannot be comfortable with them do not belong on the staff.

STRUCTURE AND MANAGEMENT

A small staff of up to a dozen true equals, well-trained and highly skilled, could function quite adequately on a basis of mutual trust, using these guidelines. They would share all work and responsibility as well as financial rewards on an equal basis. A more complex model is required in order to cope with greater demands. We recommend a detailed breakdown of duties to provide categories of staff: generalist, greeter/problem-solver, specialist, indirect service, and apprentice in any of these. Continue and strengthen an assessment/quality of service committee, an education committee, administrative committee or task force, and the committee of consultants exercising actual supervision and giving input to assessment. This combines a minimum of structure with a maximum of effectiveness.

Staff powers should be broad but limited to overall guidance. Decision-making and information exchange, both necessary functions, should be separated, with weekly staff information meetings for both administrative and guest service problems. Attendance at fifty percent of the meetings should be mandatory, and they might be rotated through the days of the week. Monthly *decision-making* meetings should be held, at which time operating policy decisions are reviewed, recommendations made to coordinators, one or two coordinators elected for six-month terms, and membership on operating committees established.

As was once the case at the Fort, three elected coordinators would be in charge of day-to-day operation, with limited rotating terms. As we now envisage it, however, the coordinators of the future should fulfill stated functions and thus meet certain qualifications. One is in charge of assessment and quality of services and should be an experienced generalist. The second is in charge of staff education and back-up and can be either a generalist or greeter. The third is in charge of day-to-day administrative services and comes from the indirect services staff. Apprentices in any category do not serve as coordinators.

The only entirely new proposal, for those who would create a similar organization, is to create an *operating* board of directors for overall guidance, basic goal-setting, long-range planning, and financial management. This board consists of four nonstaff people (former staff members are eligible), who are knowledgeable in the service areas of the center as well as in finance, management, or public relations, plus the three elected coordinators. The founder (if there is one in the way that Joel was for Fort Help) is an ex-officio member of this board, if he or she so chooses, casts only tie-breaking votes and designates anyone to act in his or her absence. The board meets monthly and provides stability and direction, as well as conducts a regular review of operations.

The basic stipend policy encourages "volunteerism" rather than "careerism" and therefore provides that no one can derive more than a stated percentage of his or her income from the organization. A suggested amount is $150 weekly or fifty percent, whichever is less. The idea is to prevent financially as well as emotionally dependent workers for whom the center becomes a haven that protects them from the realities of the outside world.

Regarding qualifications of staff members, it might be stated as Joel originally put it:

> We want people who are mature and responsible. They must be independent and able to function without much structure or supervision, but know their limits and seek help when they need it. Our staff should be open and honest and willing to share things about themselves, their lives and their work with their coworkers, and we expect them to share their knowledge freely with others who want to learn.
>
> We want people with relevant education or life experience—enough so you can begin working with people in a helping situation without further extensive training. Degrees are neither considered sufficient nor necessary. We are more interested in you as a person.
>
> We want people who feel comfortable about the problem areas we deal with. We don't expect new staff to have experience in all of them, but we don't want staff who are prejudiced against, uncomfortable with or resistant to working with people who come to us for help—alcoholics, heroin addicts, homosexuals, men, women, overweight people, minorities, etc.
>
> Some of the additional things we will be looking at will be your past training and experience in helping/counseling, ability to differentiate clearly between yourself and whatever goes on with your guests, basic empathy, high ethical standards, good communication skills, capacity to keep and manage appointments, and receptivity to consultation and criticism both from your peers and others with greater skill, experience, or training.

With a staff composed of such people, and with minimal structure as we
have outlined, we believe that it would not be necessary for another group in
the future to go through the same trial-and-error, trial-and-success process
as we did. It is not "innovative" or "creative" to refuse to learn from experience. There are always enough *new* mistakes waiting to be made!

BUILDING THE ALTERNATIVE ORGANIZATION

One thing that has become clearer to us is that there are at least two different
breeds of futuristic organization enthusiasts: those who are sincerely looking
for a better alternative to organization, and those who want no organization at
all. The latter are *alternative extremists*, for whom a total lack of structure becomes a shibboleth to which all else is sacrificed. This can be considered mas-
ochistic and self-destructive on the part of those who choose to inflict it on
themselves; when it becomes a policy imposed on unwilling others, however,
it turns into a socially destructive power-play.

As with most problems, the best measures are preventative; more careful
planning and screening (assessment) are called for. Two kinds of people
should not be accepted on the staff: those who refuse to accept a minimum of
functional authority; and those who are satisfied with their level of skill, refusing to be apprentices even when appropriate. It should be borne in mind that
one of the purposes of an intelligently administered apprenticeship system is to
train people who will, at the end of their learning period, be fully competent
and able to take their place at the side of those who have trained them. Thus,
inexperienced people are always welcome, but they will have to "work their
way up" before they can be considered first-line staff.

In a vital creative organization, if something has been tried and doesn't
work, something new should be tried. *But if that something new doesn't work
either, then it needs to be modified.* Traditional bureaucracy often produces infe-
rior and joyless work by interfering with the creativity of the workers; an alternative operation, theoretically, will produce superior work because that
creativity is released and encouraged. Most alternative organizations that had
to provide services and were unwilling to change and restructure themselves
functionally have failed, ceasing to exist within a few years from the time they
were started. There can be great problems in differentiating between creativi-
ty/innovation/artistry and anarchy/chaos, or in applying creativity to all facets of a many-sided program.

Three major problem areas in this respect emerge out of the staff answers to
a survey conducted at mid-point in our now ten-year journey: inability to separate personal matters from work; allowing incompetent people, a minority, yet
enough to become noticeable, to become counselors without adequate supervision; and the tendency to hold too many lengthy meetings. We must find ways

to avoid these particular traps while maintaining the real strengths and innovativeness of an organization of the future. Solutions to current problems cannot be found by moving backwards in time, no matter how seductive the idea. Society has become too complex for primary disorganization.

The 1970s spawned the octopus of faceless corporations run by the tight-lipped unisex person with the button-down collar, the thin travel case, the vodka gimlet eye, and above all, the M.B.A. What the corporate image has done to working conditions, human worth, elementary decency, and dignity has not been good. Business, government, and independents all need workable alternatives. The intellectual sweat shops of the computer age are as inhumane as their manual labor counterparts of more than a century ago. They have deified bigness, profit, and technology. What was designed to serve us now intends to control us.

What concerns us is not just the establishment and operation of an innovative help program, but looking at the all-important factors that attract and keep superior workers from all possible backgrounds and lifestyles. Unless great care is taken, organization building and significant work become mutually conflictual.

IMPACT ON A DREAMER

Up, down, and sideways movements have been mirrored in Joel's own changing feelings about the center he started and nurtured. In the late fall of 1975, he wrote in a private communication to long-term present and former staff members and consultants:

> After a long, varied, lonely, and draining career spent in creating many new social programs and policies, confronting government authorities, powerful industries, and professional organizations; writing, teaching, lecturing, consulting, testifying, and parenting, cumulative frustration sometimes overwhelms me. The horrors, absurdities, and hypocrisies which surround us lead me to periodic reassessments of my involvements and priorities. Further, one of the many original concepts built into our Center when I founded it was that organizations should at least consider dissolving themselves after five years of activity, a sort of starting-over concept forcing reevaluation and avoiding the common indefinite self-perpetuation, time-wasting, and money-squandering which displace the original constructive and idealistic goals.

> There have been many satisfactions for me, most of them abstract, in the ten years since I evolved the concepts embodied in FORT HELP, first in the S.F. Health Department's Center for Special Problems which I started in 1965, and in the last five years the far more revolutionary National Center for Solving Special Social & Health Problems. These satisfactions include the help provided to many thousands with drug, sex, suicide, and other prob-

lems, face to face and by phone; the blending on our staff with equality, women and men, young and old, homosexual and heterosexual, professional and nonprofessional, paid and unpaid without medical or bureaucratic hierarchies; independence of government and the media; training hundreds who have gone on to other programs; demonstration of new approaches which, in part, have been taken up by many agencies and individuals in the United States and abroad.

My dissatisfactions include our failure to attract and our driving away outstanding staff members and people needing help of diverse ages, lifestyles, races, and economic levels; the preoccupation of many staff with the mental health model of clients-patients, psychotherapy maintenance, individual rather than group counseling, emphasis on weakness and dependence rather than strength and health, and a failure to develop the eclectic blend of growth techniques, new and old approaches which I had envisaged; insufficient attention to our sex and drug programs; lack of fundraising whether it be seeking out individual donors, foundation grants, a broader range of guests (people coming for help), or even the simple sale (or rental) of the film, buttons, bumperstickers, and books I have made available; an inflexible and hypocritical stipend-salary policy which is unworkable and has lost us many good staff members; and too many time-consuming, unproductive meetings which, like many things organizations attempt to do, are anachronisms and where people take themselves too seriously while failing to give enough decentralized authority to work (task) groups (committees) which are capable of doing it quicker and better.

Possible alternative future plans: 1) dissolve the Center; 2) set up 2 or more teams with different rules and practices, one perhaps including many of the present staff doing things they like to do, another returning former staff and new people either focusing on other approaches to problem-solving or on consulting, training, preventive checkups, 24-hour telephone line, self-development seminars for the public, or other valuable and interesting activities --- these teams operating semiautonomously and responsible for their own funding under the general rubric of our state licensing, federal tax-exemption, Board of Advisors, etc.; 3) continuing as is with my leaving but helping you as individuals and as a group to advance your careers (in the same way I have in the past) and to fill my legal, medical, community, and other roles; 4) other ideas to be suggested by you in writing.

He eventually chose a combination of 2) and 3), diversifying and decreasing his involvement at the center. The departure of those staff members with whom he had worked most closely, the achievement of many of the original goals including shared leadership not dependent on him, and the devastating effects of the legal and media attack combined to reduce his association to occasional consulting and to service on the board of directors.

RENEWING ORGANIZATIONS

For there to be civilized organizations and societies, all existing organizations—academic, professional, service, business, and independent—can profit from a reexamination of their practices, goals, and regulations, followed by a discarding of what is outmoded and harmful, and by adoption of new, human, and efficient policies. As part of this, staff members-employees-managers, ideally all co-owners or co-leaders, should meet regularly for specific and time-limited discussion on how to do the work better and help people more, to praise those doing well, to hold accountable those doing poorly, and to make their work relevant and satisfying. Fellow employee-owners should vote on raises, promotions, and other key decisions. All officials-administrators should spend at least a day a week doing line work or direct services. Everyone from top to bottom should share in all profits and rewards of the group effort, thereby replacing the traditional labor-management adversarial relationship—the *we* versus *they* ideology—with shared responsibility and authority.

We have proven that new ideas/concepts/approaches, even when ambitious and complex, can attract large numbers of people and can survive for many years. There is considerable latent altruism to be developed among a significant minority of people who want to live a truly religious and saintly life as "born again" humans rather than following the perversions of Christianity and Americanism that we see around us.

We see other helping organizations as having government funding and control, a salaried administrative hierarchy, medical-physician elitism, a discriminatory white and "hip" orientation, rapid turnover of staff, overprescribing of drugs, little supervision or quality control, few patients' rights, gearing priorities to where the money is, and no equality for paid versus unpaid/volunteer staff. We see ourselves as having a more relaxed atmosphere, less filling out of forms, greater acceptance of a broader range of patients, and the provision of more time for talking with the patient.

THE FUTURE

If we could substitute a narrow rear-view mirror of the world for a panoramic forward view, we would see increasing discontent and alienation, and decreased productivity, among the work forces of government, civil and military, business and nonprofit organizations. We see disputes, strikes, violence, absenteeism, accidents, drug abuse, especially alcoholism and cigarette smoking, psychosomatic illnesses, and a high divorce rate. We have massive underemployment, unemployment, and successful affirmative action only for the ethically and mentally handicapped. Sometimes overwhelming structural barriers have been imposed by organizational administrators in medicine, psychiatry and other fields, and by the many powerful special interest groups.

Bureaucracy is indispensable as an instrument of power for those who head it. This power is too often used for self-aggrandisement and perpetuation of the status quo rather than for progress. One negative aspect of alternative or counterorganizations is that they take the pressure off such groups as health and mental health departments, instead of increasing the pressure to reform them. They also help to establish and institutionalize a two-tiered system of care. Such inequities as verbal facility, going to the right schools, self-confidence (if not arrogance), and differing levels of attraction to power, further impede our efforts to make organizations responsive and adaptive rather than oligarchical and totalitarian (fascist/communist). Our leaders are now caretakers and entertainers, using others' ideas and speeches while subservient to special interests in and out of government, to the polls, and to the media. We have a society of mini-societies out to "get theirs."

Both a cosmic scale emphasizing the relative smallness and lack of civilization of humans, and a human scale stressing individual identity, ethics, and social justice, are needed by those who want to create, work in, and be served by better organizations/institutions. Most likely we will continue into the next century with various types of organizations coexisting at different stages of development: some centralized and some decentralized; some with conventional bureaucratic leadership and some with democratic-inspirational-facilitative leadership; and some encouraging participation of those coming for services. More people will have pluralistic commitments to a number of organizations during the same periods of their work lives. Good men and women will continue to be difficult to find for the most responsible jobs because they have been exhausted by their legitimate quest for organizational utopia. They are not prepared to sell out, be co-opted, or to engage in the lies and manipulations that are part of conventional organizational success.

Among a growing minority of staff members-workers-employees-civil servants, the trend will be toward job-sharing, flexi-scheduling, a three or four day week, no tenure or seniority, sabbaticals of several months duration every few years, rotated leadership, autonomous work teams, encouraged reporting of abuses and incompetence, new kinds of unions with voluntary membership (open shop), work at home using the latest telephone and computer technology, robots for menial and backbreaking work, de-professionalizing and de-mythologizing of expertise, regionalization and decentralization, and emphasis on service to others. Respect will not be based on personal power over others, but rather everyone's interests will be seen as identical with a more even distribution of responsibility. Smaller groups, rather than large public assemblies, will do the decision making, and, in general, much more extensive use will be made of our knowledge of group process, a blending of the usually separate fields of organizational behavior, public administration, social psychology, and group therapy. Books such as this one will hopefully dispel the historical tendency of newly developing institutions failing to learn from their predecessors.

THE ROLE OF FORT HELP

We, like other innovative organizations, believe that we provided care for people who had nowhere to turn—the outlaws, outcasts, strangers, and scapegoats of society, as well as for ordinary people who had alternatives but were seeking something better. We provided many with their first jobs and with important new careers. We trained people to overcome obstacles and to engage in participatory democracy, as difficult as it was and is. We provided a community or family for the lonely and alienated. Fort Help was and is a living witness to desired shifts: to best, not most; to interdependence and independence, not dependence; to harmony, not mastery; to cooperation, not competition; to development of people, not organizations; to democracy, not totalitarianism; to decentralization, not centralization; to work as fulfilling and purposeful, not demeaning; and to consultation, not arbitrary and irrational authority.

Our main contribution was to be witnesses, exemplars, prophets, antibureaucrats, and antitotalitarians in a world we never made but had to live in. We shared in the development of new ways of living and working, showed resourcefulness and perseverance, became polymaths, and tried to put into practice the ideas and ideals expressed by Jesus, Marx, and other venerated, but not emulated, leaders. There was equality without the barriers of age and sex, and involvement or engagement as the antidote to "me" organizations.

Edith Hamilton, in her classic works on ancient Greece, brought out that the quality the Greeks valued most was sophrosune, a concept combining the qualities of self-control, knowing oneself, doing nothing to excess, harmony, and excellence. A voluntary obedience to unenforceable laws, such as kindness, compassion, and unselfishness, was considered a basic aspect of freedom without which life would be intolerable.

The social artistry exhibited in the creation of new organizations to meet human needs is little rewarded. Many creative tasks are ephemeral, from cooking a good meal to parenthood; and tens of thousands of people throughout our country are engaged in saintly, altruistic, or social reform activities which go unrecognized. As we did at Fort Help, they are putting forth excellence as a counter to society's progressive mediocrity, and they are showing that precedent is no consideration, that new ideas can be put into immediate operation. There are the talkers versus the doers, and there are the passive, uncivil, and abrasive rather than those legitimately impatient, independent, direct, and constructive.

In some ways, it is a revolutionary idea that individuals or groups can solve their own problems; that short-term, independence-oriented help can substitute for dependence, dropping out, and failure; that people can be responded to as guests, friends, or students rather than as objects or numbers; and that organizations can be worthwhile even if they exist for no more than five years, as ad hoc, voluntary, goal-oriented groupings of people. Other people's dreams and revolutions can be broader or more restrictive than ours. Our example is not intended to be followed literally or fully. The true leader is a realizer of dreams.

Together, we need to engage in a brick-by-brick rebuilding of society, starting with ourselves, our families, our organizations, our neighborhoods, our cities, and our country. We need to do this from the bottom up rather than the top down, in the way that artisans build cohesive and inspirational symbols.

The original Olympic ideal, although lost in the current nationalism and competitiveness, was: "Ask not for victory, ask for courage, for if you can endure the struggle you bring honor to us all." We need other successful models of alternative organizations like Fort Help to constructively channel the anger and energy of modern society toward solution of our many problems. Let us begin.

A DOMAIN-THEORY ANALYSIS OF THE FORT HELP EXPERIENCE

Paul R. Mico and James M. Kouzes

The uniqueness of the Fort Help, community-based, alternative-organization experience lies in the great emphasis that a group of service-delivery colleagues placed on running their own show, and in the fact that they have been doing it for the past ten years. From our perspective, they accentuated the role of the service-delivery component and minimized the role to be played by two other important components of public service organizations—management, and policy-making boards of directors. In this regard, their experience is an important contribution to a better understanding of organizational behavior, especially when viewed from the context of our *Domain Theory*. What we propose to do in the analytical chapter of this book is to introduce Domain Theory and then apply it to the Fort Help experience.

AN INTRODUCTION TO DOMAIN THEORY

It is a fundamental American principle that human services should be planned and controlled by the people for whom they are intended. As implemented, this notion has helped to account for the phenomenon of community-based organizations. The purpose of this chapter is to provide a point of view regarding the behavior of these organizations; the idea is that such a view might enable organizational leaders such as Dr. Joel Fort and Mr. Lothar Salin to help theirs operate more effectively.

Community-based organizations, as we ordinarily know them, are composed of *governing bodies* and *staff*. *Governing bodies*, or boards, can be thought of as either public or private. Public bodies tend to be governmental in nature, established by law and mandated to serve public needs. Private bodies are voluntary, established by groups of people who share common concerns and who propose to meet specific needs. In both cases, generally, members are elected or appointed to them by a specifically defined public, known as a constituency. Board members are responsible to their constituencies; they serve specific terms of office; they receive no pay. They are volunteers.

Members of *staffs*, on the other hand, tend to be paid employees. They are hired for their professional or technical expertise, for indefinite periods of time. They tend to be regarded either as part of *administration* or of *program*. *Administration* consists of management and such related support services as finance, budgeting, personnel, data processing, secretarial, and maintenance. *Program* consists of those professional and material resources which combine to provide the organization's services to its clients, or "guests," as the authors of the book prefer.

The Dominant Paradigm of Organizational Behavior

It is the dominant view[1] regarding the behavior of organizations that the people who make them up serve common goals. They take certain resources, such as money, personnel, equipment, supplies, and facilities, and transform these into the products and services delivered to their clients. In order to do this, they organize themselves into specialized units of professional or technical expertise, and use a variety of rational procedures and systems to produce and deliver their services. The purpose of management is to control and coordinate the entire process so that it can perform smoothly and successfully. Success is measured by productivity and by the cost effectiveness of the services provided. This dominant view and its theoretical formulations evolved out of the study of business and industrial organizations (see Figure 1). It is taught in management schools, and provides the basis for the current practice of planned organizational change, better known as Organization Development.[2-4]

We Don't Work That Way

But human service organizations do not function the way that the dominant model says they should, as those who work in and with them will testify. The following composite descriptions are examples of behaviors that cause us to raise questions.

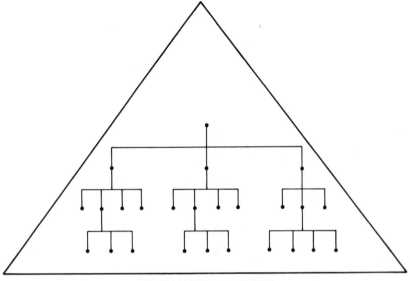

MANAGEMENT DOMAIN

Principles: Hierarchical control and coordination
Success measures: Cost efficiency effectiveness
Structure: Bureaucratic
Work modes: Use of linear techniques and tools

FIGURE 1

At the Governing Body level   Not all board members are clear about the
basic mission of their organization. There is disagreement about the approaches thought best to take with clientele: some favor the dominant liberal
view of "work with them and give them more"; others believe that clients "get
away with too much" and should be held more accountable. Policy makers do
not understand why the program staff seems unable to make much of a dent in
the problem being served. They feel pressured by their constituencies to show
success and keep costs down. Not all policy makers understand what policy is
and how to make it; not all have adequate skills in being an effective board
member. Some policy makers feel that they are "rubberstamps" for the staff,
that the staff makes the important decisions and then strategizes about how to
get the board to accept them. Others feel that the staff is their basic tool for
carrying out their directions, and should be controlled more tightly than they
are. Policy makers complain about having too much homework to do, too

many reports to read. They resent being presented with voluminous reports when they come to their meetings, and then being expected to make important decisions regarding those reports without having had adequate opportunity to understand them. Under the surface, the members of the governing body do not feel appreciated by staff for the large amounts of volunteer time and energies they give. They feel accountable for what the organization does but have little sense of the control of it.

At the management level   The managers have several concerns. They believe that the board interferes too much with their day-to-day operations; that it does not have an adequate understanding of the problems and of the management data base needed to make constructive policy decisions; that it is erratic in its actions and too time-consuming in its deliberations; that it is too easily influenced by special interest groups; that it is not as committed to the organization's cause as they, the managers, are. They believe that the program staff is too resistant to the use of more efficient or productive methods for the handling of clients and case loads; that staff gets too involved or "hung up" with their clients; that staff does not support, or conform to, the basic rules or norms of how the organization should operate. They, the managers, believe that the ultimate responsibility for the success or failure of the organization is theirs, and that they do not get enough resources or support to discharge this responsibility adequately.

At the program staff level   Program personnel perceive themselves as the "front lines" of the organization. They believe that neither management nor board really understands what they do, or trusts them in doing it; that the quality of their work must give way to the pressures on them to produce; that the work they do requires flexibility in approaches and work periods, not conformity to rigid procedures and schedules; that there is too little power or influence for them in the organization's policy making or allocation of resources; that there is too much paperwork to do, too many rules and procedures to follow, and too little opportunity to experience creativity or success in their work.

What Makes Us Tick? Domain Theory

What is happening? Do the composite experiences above suggest that human services organizations (HSOs) behave differently than the dominant view has taught us? Or is it that the dominant view is still appropriate, but that the problems described are more "personality conflicts" and "poor communications" than they are structural?

Our view, based on our studies and experiences, is that HSOs are different.[5] Further, these differences have important implications for both the theory of organizational behavior and the practice of organization development. We are not alone. Other researchers have reported on the distinctive attributes of HSOs[6-10] as well.

We trace the origins of our theoretical work back to 1974. We were engaged in a project to train a group of HSO management teams who were dealing with problems involving interagency health and welfare integration of services. During the program, we became acutely aware of the different points of view which policy makers, managers, and service deliverers hold about the same issues. The following year, we designed a project to develop these three different levels. Agencies had to designate special teams from each level in order to participate in the training. Out of this experience came additional insights regarding the uniqueness of each level, and of the tensions between and among them. These ideas were further tested and refined in a three-year demonstration project involving eight mental health organizations, funded by the National Institutes of Mental Health.

We later called these levels "domains," defining this term to mean "a sphere of influence or control claimed by a social entity." We see HSOs as consisting of three distinct domains—Policy, Management, and Service. Each functions by a set of governing principles, success measures, structural arrangements, and work modes or technologies, such as characterized by the dominant paradigm (Figure 1). The difference is that each domain in an HSO operates differently, each is in contrast with the others. The result is an organization which is in a constant state of tension, caused by the push and pull of domains that are incompatible with each other, thereby producing discordance and conflict (see Figure 2). What holds the domains together in an HSO is a unique purpose to which most members subscribe, as well as a set of legal-economic agreements which give it viability.

Policy Domain   The governing body or board of directors' level of the organization is the one accorded the role of formulating policies and directions. Typically, it is composed of elected or appointed representatives who have a public constituency of one kind or another to whom they feel accountable. It is this constituency and this sense of accountability that provides the Policy Domain with one of its basic principles, legitimacy by the consent of the governed. The other principles include: membership participation on the basis of "one-person, one-vote"; a structure based on representation; work modes involving the uses of negotiating, bargaining and voting; and measures of success on the basis of equity, or impartial and fair policy decisions for themselves and their constituencies.

Management Domain   Management in HSOs follows the dominant paradigm. It attempts to mirror the model of business and industrial management. Its governing principles are: legitimacy by technical expertise; hierarchical control and coordination; a structure based on bureaucratized units of resources; work modes utilizing such linear tools and procedures as management-by-objectives, zero-based budgeting, and management-information systems; and success based on productivity and cost efficiency.

THE ELECTORATE

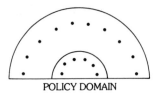

POLICY DOMAIN

Principles: Consent of the governed
Success measures: Equity
Structure: Representative participative
Work modes: Voting, bargaining, negotiating

Discordance   Disjunction   Conflict

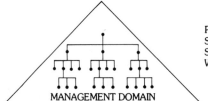

MANAGEMENT DOMAIN

Principles: Hierarchical control and coordination
Success measures: Cost efficiency effectiveness
Structure: Bureaucratic
Work modes: Use of linear techniques and tools

Discordance   Disjunction   Conflict

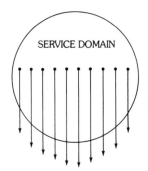

SERVICE DOMAIN

Principles: Autonomy, self-regulation
Success measures: Quality of service
                              Good standards of practice
Structure: Collegial
Work modes: Client-specific
                        Problem solving

FIGURE 2

Service Domain   The professionals who make up the program, or service delivery, domain generally have a background of many years of study,
training, and experience. They see themselves as "professional," possessing the
expertise to respond to the needs and demands of their clients, and having the
values and ethics needed for self governance. Their governing principles are:

legitimacy by professional expertise; the reliance on autonomy and self regulation; the preference for collegial, team-like structures; the use of client-oriented problem solving methods which are adaptable to various contingencies; and success based on the quality of care provided to the client, or the personal satisfaction of having lived up to one's professional standards.

Tensions and Contentions

The very principles or qualities that serve to give domains their unique identities and enable them to function appropriately serve also to place them in contention with each other. The very sense of separate identities, if nothing else, creates tension and distance between and among the three domains. It makes difficult the development and preservation of a shared common vision or mission among the three. Often, it seems, the three domains are moving in different directions. The tensions that are created involve contrasting principles, different rhythms of change, power and control, and limited domain capacities.

The Tension of Contrasting Principles   The Policy Domain derives its legitimacy from the consent of its constituency, or governed. This contrasts sharply with Management's legitimacy by technical expertise and Service's legitimacy by professional expertise. When legitimacy is an issue, the conflict can be sharp. There is tension between the principle of one-person one-vote, which characterizes the Policy Domain, with those of Management's hierarchical control and coordination, and Service's autonomy and self regulation. Policy's representative, participative structure contrasts with Management's bureaucratic and Service's collegial preferences. Policy's uses of negotiating, bargaining, and voting contrasts with Management's linear tools and Service's client-oriented, contingency problem solving. Finally, Policy's reliance on the success measures of equity differ significantly from Management's productivity and cost effectiveness, and from Service's quality of service or the application of professional standards.

The Tension of Different Change Rhythms   The drum beat of change is different for each domain. The Policy Domain must be responsive to its political environment. Change, there, is cyclical, dependent on the outcome of the next two- or four-year election, when new forces may be brought into power or incumbent forces retained. For the community-based organization, the political issue may be repeated annually, when a third of its board members' terms expire and the chance to put some "new blood" on it is presented. For the Management Domain, the rhythm is both economic and technologic: economic, ranging from annual organizational budget cycles, to broader issues of inflation and money markets; technologic, in terms of the rapid developments affecting data processing and other linear procedures, as well as the basic roles and functions of the personnel who handle them. For the Service Domain, the rhythm of change is long range: the causes of the problems which bring the clients and the program professionals together sometimes can barely be altered from one generation to another, since they may require years of intensive social problem solving, involving large macrosystem efforts; in addition, changes in the professionals' preparation and practice fields are slow. Finally, what the managers may believe to be a good strategy for the development of the organization may not be politically expedient from the policy perspective, and may be very disruptive to the program efforts of the professionals.

The Tension of Power and Control   In the business and industrial world, managers have powerful discretionary uses of rewards, structural arrangements, information processes, leadership initiatives, and task assignments, which enable them to maintain a high degree of control over their organizations. In HSO's, the situation is different. The Management Domain is accountable to the Policy Domain, supposedly, but nevertheless may attempt to impose its will on its governing body by formulating policies itself, by withholding information on other decision options, or by intimidating the body members with technical and professional expertise. Managers exert dominance over the Service Domain by controlling budget data and rewards, and by enforcing conformity to the linear management tools which the professionals find irrelevant and time consuming. The Policy Domain exerts its control over the Management Domain by the exercise of hiring-and-firing authority over the top managers, by approving or fixing the budget, by accepting or rejecting reports, and by the close monitoring of day-to-day management operations. The Service Domain exercises its power by resisting the demands of the managers or policy makers, by the use or threat of strike, by members who bypass management and take their needs or demands directly to sympathetic policy makers, and by having their power needs fulfilled through unions or employee associations.

The Tension of Limited Domain Capacities   There is nothing that equips a new member of a policy board or management group with an automatic understanding of the principles that characterize the domain that he or she has joined, so that he or she can perform effectively in the required role. Members of a Policy Domain are volunteers, and not always experienced in serving on other governing bodies. They may be managers or program professionals of other organizations, and bring those domain perspectives to the policy body. Managers of HSOs rarely are trained formally for their roles, unlike business or industrial managers who have their "MBA union cards." Usually, they are program professionals who move up into management because of preference or, more likely, for the higher salaries and status not available to them as service deliverers. If any domain approaches the desired state of having its members understand its operating principles, it is the Service Domain, particularly if the personnel are professionally trained. These principles are modeled by their university instructors (who are part of the Service Domain in their own academic organizations) and are promoted by their professional associations (whose values are Service-Domain related). But it is not always that simple for the Service Domain: many organizations use volunteers or nonprofessionals to deliver services who have not had the advantage of academic values training for their domain roles (as was the case at Fort Help).

DOMAIN THEORY APPLIED TO FORT HELP

As already suggested, Fort Help was intended to be a *Service-Domain* organization, exclusively. A board of directors was created only because it was required as a part of the legal incorporation necessary for nonprofit, tax-exempt status. The board's role was established to be advisory rather than for policy making, and for help in fund raising and publicity. It was kept at an arm's distance throughout the experience. For all intents and purposes, Dr. Fort created the basic mission and policies for the organization.

The effort to prevent a management locus of influence from forming was a conscious strategy from the beginning. *Management* was equated with *bureaucracy* and Dr. Fort's negative experiences with bureaucracy had resulted in his determination that Fort Help would never become bureaucratic. Therefore, management-type decision making, supervision, and coordination were handled on a collegial-consensus basis rather than hierarchically—until a staff revolt threatened to change the nature of the organization, and Dr. Fort had to intervene as the manager. The use of such management tools as budgeting, billing and collections, cost accounting, fee setting, and service statistics were accorded low-priority status—task responsibilities to be avoided, interferences with the preoccupation of services to guests—until the Medi-Cal legal-financial crisis hit the organization and almost destroyed it.

What evolves, then, is a classic case study of a Service-Domain organization which placed high emphasis on the following domain principles:

1. A competency-based rather than credential-based determinant of staff capability.

2. Peer review as the basis for improving both competency and quality of care.

3. Collegial (team) work groupings.

4. Consensus decision making, with some representation-type decision making structures.

5. Autonomy and self regulation.

Discussion

We have several observations and thoughts about the Fort Help experience, viewed from the Service-Domain perspective.

A single domain HSO Can a single-domain organization survive and provide human services effectively in today's turbulent, complex society? The answer is yes, as Fort Help has demonstrated, but under certain conditions. It would have to be free of legal and financial accountability. For example, Dr. Fort and Mr. Salin speculate that the reason they were not able to obtain foundation grants was because they could not convince the foundations that they were well managed and responsible.

To really get by without a Policy Domain requires some process whereby the service deliverers are able to stay in close touch with constituents and clients alike. Fort Help was battered by its environment—by advocacy groups, regulatory agencies, stakeholder funding agencies, governmental counterparts, media (when it got in trouble), and clients who coalesced with dissident staff to try to gain control of the organization. A properly designed Policy Domain develops and maintains effective linkages with these external forces, helping to bring relevancy and stability to the organization. This linking would have to be done by the service deliverers. The Fort Help personnel did not do this—they concentrated on serving their guests. Only Dr. Fort, it seemed, dealt with these external forces, and most often on a reactive basis (after a problem had developed) rather than a proactive, prevention-oriented basis. It is interesting to note that Dr. Fort and Mr. Salin conclude that the one thing they would do differently would be to create an operating board of directors.

To really get by without a Management Domain requires that the basic management functions be conducted, anyway, without the existence of a "domain force," as such. Two options seem obvious: one, service deliverers should learn how to use necessary management tools, and agree to share the responsibilities equitably; or, two, a contract should be let to an external person or firm to provide this function for the organization. What is even more important is that a basic *positive value* would have to be inculcated into the behavioral processes of the service deliverers—that good management is also good service delivery. At Fort Help, management as a negative value was a dominant norm.

Competency-based performance One of the important learnings from Fort Help was the way by which competency-based performance began to be developed and refined. Levels of competency were established, with clear indications of how one could move upward from one level to another. The concept of apprenticeship was established, heavy emphasis was placed on training, and excellent peer review processes became an integral part of the collegial operations. This latter point is significant. There is a myth that human service professionals value peer review as a standard-maintaining process. Our experience with HSOs suggests, in fact, that peer review is a highly threatening process and that efforts to introduce it are usually unsuccessful. Fort Help is an example of how it can be institutionalized and used productively.

Coping with dissident staff Some of the more eloquent parts of this book are the insights garnered from the types of personnel attracted to alternative organizations, and how to cope with them. Dissidents almost won their revolution to take control of Fort Help at one time, and a strong self-interest group almost changed the mission of it at another. The insights are: awareness that stringent selection is essential to the recruitment of personnel whose primary motivation is to help other people rather than to meet their own needs; and that "weeding out" of those who are not able to demonstrate that motivation may be necessary from time to time. Unfortunately, few bureaucratic organizations can control either process very effectively.

Rewards A basic value at Fort Help was the notion of equal rewards (stipends) for all. Although the financial remuneration was low, the fact that the value was emphasized prevented what might otherwise have been a serious problem—conflict over perceived inequities in pay. Since there was no higher pay established for managerial work, no one felt the need to give up the satisfaction of one task in order to gain more money for doing another one not as satisfying. What comes through the experience is the sense of *task satisfaction* as the basic reward which Fort Helpers wanted and received—they liked what they were doing, and left only when they found a more satisfying job or were forced to seek a better salary elsewhere.

CONCLUSION

Fort Help, from an organizational-behavior point of view, is a testimony to the functioning of a Service Domain. It has lessons for every human service organization, if for no other reason than to arrive at a better understanding of this one domain. It is essential reading for others who would create single Service-Domain, alternative organizations. It suggests what strengths can be emphasized and what problems avoided. In addition, Domain Theory serves to explain the properties that are essential for a well-functioning domain. The better that staff can understand and utilize those properties, the more successful they should be in what they are trying to do.

REFERENCES

1. Trist, E. "Collaboration in Work Settings: A Personal Perspective." *Journal of Applied Behavioral Science*, 1977, *13* (3), 268-278.

2. French, W. L., and Bell, C. H. Jr. *Organization Development: Behavioral Science Interventions for Organization Improvement.* Englewood Cliffs, NJ: Prentice-Hall, 1973.

3. Huse, E. F. *Organization Development and Change.* St. Paul, MN: West Publishing, 1975.

4. Schmuck, R. A., and Miles, M. B. *Organization Development in Schools.* Palo Alto, CA: Mayfield Press (formerly National Press Books), 1971.

5. Kouzes, J. M., and Mico, P. R. "Domain Theory: An Introduction to Organizational Behavior in Human Service Organizations." *Journal of Applied Behavioral Science*, 1979, Nov.-Dec., 449-469. Also, P. R. Mico and J. M. Kouzes "What Makes Us Run? Domain Theory Applied to Youth Service Organizations." *New Designs for Youth Development* (5), no. 5, 1980, 1-5.

6. Harshbarger, D. "The Human Service Organization." in H. W. Demone, Jr. & Dr. Harshbarger (Eds.), *A Handbook of Human Service Organizations.* New York: Behavioral Publications, 1974.

7. Hasenfeld, Y., and English, R. A. "Human Service Organizations: A Conceptual Overview." in Y. Hasenfeld & R. A. English (Eds.), *Human Service Organizations.* Ann Arbor: The University of Michigan Press, 1974.

8. Weisbord, M.R. "Why Organization Development Hasn't Worked (so far) in Medical Centers." *Health Care Management Review*, 1976, *1* (Spring), 17-28.

9. Jacques, E. A. *A General Theory of Bureaucracy.* New York: Halsted Press, 1976.

10. Weick, K. E. "Educational Organizations as Loosely Coupled Systems." *Administrative Science Quarterly*, 1976, *21* (1), 1-19.

REASONS FOR WORKING AT FORT HELP

1. Wanted to explore something that was different from the clinical setting of my training.

2. Had worked for and admired Joel Fort, wanted to make Fort Help a success.

3. Field placement that was related to alternative humanistic counseling.

4. Wanted a place where therapy was based on values and ways of seeing people and the world similar to mine. . .a place to learn more.

COUNSELING AREAS

Drug abuse

Crime and delinquency

Violence and uncontrollable rage or hatred

Compulsive gambling

Suicide

Death and dying

Chronic debts and inability to manage finances

Overweight (obesity)

Insomnia

Unfulfilled potential and problems of identity and alienation

Sex-related problems

In our effort to treat sexual unhappiness and inadequacy, we do not attempt to *change* anyone's sexual orientation to fit prevalent values. Rather, we hope to help each person to be happier, more competent, and more fulfilled with the sexual identity and life style that has been chosen.

NEWSLETTER

A Program of and for the Future: My Vision of the Center for Solving Special Social and Health Problems (Joel Fort, 1970)

Evolving partially from related programs (the San Francisco Health Department's Center for Special Problems; the Mobile Health and Welfare (HELP) Unit; the National Sex and Drug Forum; and the Police-Revolutionary workshops) that I originated over the past five years, and partially from my diverse life experiences, training, and crusades for social reform, this Center has been steadily developing over the past year. Its direction has been greatly influenced by the gratifying and impressive commitment of about one hundred highly talented and knowledgeable people of varying backgrounds who have joined its staff. As we gradually phase in our pioneering and ambitious program—that is, to help people with drug, sex, and other special problems; to train others and receive training; to complete the construction and decoration of our space; to raise money; etc.—we are being paid to the satisfaction of direct constructive participation in solving some of the most serious and pervasive problems of our age, while also making our lives meaningful and relevant. The Center, or colloquially Fort Help, represents many important things for our present and for our future. We are to provide:

1. Badly needed special long-term services to those with drug (alcohol, tobacco, pills, LSD, narcotics), or sex (homosexual, heterosexual, or transsexual) problems; to the suicidal and dying; to insomniacs and those who are overweight; and to problems of crime and violence. Ours is the only facility anywhere to have the emphasis of seeking social health rather than a simplistic narrow concept of mental health.

2. The most eclectic and innovative helping facility anywhere— blending every traditional and new technique from psychotherapy

and encounter groups to hypnosis, massage, and music provided by professional and nonprofessional helpers selected solely for competency, commitment, and maturity (including altruism) rather than for their degrees, old age, or conformity.

3. A new model of health care—accessible, human, oriented to keeping people well, open to all, irrespective of ability to pay, comprehensive, and a maximum use of paraprofessionals.

4. A new organizational style—a voluntary association of people dedicated to solving problems in a non-hierarchical, non-authoritarian, status-free manner—a parallel institution doing privately and urgently without profit what needs to be done and without bureaucratic buck-passing, inefficiency and dehumanization.

5. A bridge over the increasing fragmentation of American society. Rather than exploiting separate groups such as "hippies," blacks, the middle class, one neighborhood, we are reaching out to everyone who has problems that can be helped. Insofar as possible, ours is a regional and national program analogous in its fields to those of the Mayo and Menninger clinics.

6. A clinic that eliminates the pathological frame of reference, labeling, and stigmatizing—where staff relate to those who come for help as individual human beings seeking aid for one area of their life and receiving it from an interdisciplinary, eclectic staff of greeters, problem-solvers, helpers, and culture workers, rather than from the possibly more limited psychiatrist, psychologist, or social worker.

7. A social movement and crusade seeking to involve people, provide positive alternatives, change society constructively, and enhance human potential—as well as solve particular problems.

8. A research, educational, and training center.

9. A demonstration project that should be a model for cities in this country and abroad.

10. A place where values, ethics, idealism, and consistency of words and actions are stressed, where we try to live according to what we believe in and provide reality instead of public relations imagery, where we pursue excellence and seek mutual tolerance for different lifestyles.

APPENDIX D
ON NOT SMOKING

1. Please respect the right of non-smokers, including children, to *breathe clean air* and limit your smoking to consenting adults in private. We have determined that public smoking of tobacco (or marijuana) is harmful.

2. Tobacco contains a drug (nicotine) and a poison gas consisting of carbon monoxide, arsenic, cyanide, coal tars, formaldehyde, etc. It is one of our two biggest drug abuse problems, causing 400,000 deaths per year in the U.S. alone (from heart attacks, cancer, strokes, bronchitis, and fires). Death cures smoking and is nature's way of changing our habits.

3. By not smoking you'll live longer; save money; be healthier; reduce burns, fire, and air pollution; have a better sex life; smell and eat better; and help others.

4. Thank you for **NOT SMOKING**.

(From *Breathe Free*, the Stop Smoking Program of the National Center for Solving Special Social and Health Problems, Fort Help, 169 Eleventh St., San Francisco, California 94103)

APPENDIX E
DIET

1. Concentrate on fish, meats, vegetables, and plenty of liquids.

2. Fruit is good also and often can satisfy the urge for sugar. Watch how much of it you eat though and stay away from bananas, cherries, watermelon, dried fruits, grapes, papayas, and mangos.

3. Fish is very healthy because of its low cholesterol content; experts suggest trying to eat more fish than meat. When preparing meat or fish, broil, pan broil, bake or roast it—do not fry!

4. Cut down on carbohydrates as much as possible and limit yourself to one or two slices of bread a day; eliminate altogether crackers, cookies, desserts, etc.

5. Cook eggs in shell or poach or scramble (without fat).

6. Remember that it is the total caloric value you take in each day that determines whether you gain or lose—in other words, what you eat altogether in a given day. If, for example, you were to eat nothing but some fish and a few vegetables all day, but had fourteen pieces of fudge while watching the late news on television lying in bed that night, you would gain weight.

7. There are a great variety of vegetables, fish, and meats. Try to vary your eating—this helps you feel less *deprived* and makes meals more enjoyable. Remember, the goal is not to deprive yourself of the joy of eating; this is a pleasure in life you will always keep, hopefully.

8. Try to eat *only when you are truly hungry*. This may be three to several times a day. Many people prefer several small meals or nibbling to a set schedule of breakfast, lunch at noon, and dinner at 6:00. Many compulsive eaters rarely, if ever, feel truly hungry—they haven't waited long enough between eating periods to feel this. Compulsive eating is often due to more complex reasons than hunger. Try and become aware of what you are *feeling when* you get an urge to eat—is it hunger or is it some other feeling?

Many people *block out the amount* of food they are eating as well as their feelings when eating; guilt feelings result later from the realization that they've overeaten. Try *not* to block out and *not* to feel guilty about food—rather try and to concentrate exactly on your motives and goals.

9. Concentrate on eating *slowly* and *really tasting* each bite of food.

10. Concentrate on one day at a time rather than worrying about the entire ten weeks.

11. Weigh yourself *only once a week*—preferably in the morning (when you get up) and preferably on Wednesday. We will keep a record of your weight each week.

12. Please keep a written record (food diary) of what you eat each day and when. Write it down at the end of each evening or the next morning. This will help you to become *aware* of your eating habits and also will provide us with material for group sessions.

AMMUNITION FOODS

Eat all you want!

asparagus	dandelion greens	string beans
bean sprouts	endive	summer squash
beets (and greens)	escarole	tea, coffee
broccoli	green & red peppers	tomato juice
Brussels sprouts	kale	unflavored gelatin
cabbage	leeks	vinegar and
cauliflower	lettuce	wine vinegar
celery	mushrooms	water
chard	mustard greens	
cucumbers	onions	
bouillon	parsley	
carbonated beverages	pimentos	
(low calorie)	pickles	
herbs and spices	radishes	
horseradish	rhubarb	
lemons, limes	sauerkraut	
mustard	soy sauce	
seltzer	spinach	

COMFORTING FOODS

These are relatively low calorie and more filling than ammunition foods. They are great for fighting off that urge, and to calm cravings.

apples	cottage cheese	scallops
apricots	eggplant	shrimp
artichokes	grapefruit	strawberries
cantalope	lean beefburgers	tangerines
carrots	lobster	tomatoes
chestnuts	mussels	veal
chicken	pears	

"POISON" FOODS

Stay away from these altogether

alcoholic beverages	fat meats
avocado	gravies, honey
bacon	griddle cakes
baked beans	ice cream, malted milk
butter, cream cheese	jams, jellies
cake, candy, chocolate	macaroni, mayonnaise
cereals, corn	muffins, biscuits
cookies, crackers	nuts, oil, olives
cream, creamed soups	pancakes, peanut butter
dates	potatoes
doughnuts	pie, popcorn, chips
dressings (except vinegar)	pretzels, pudding
dried fruits	pizza, spaghetti
french fries, fried foods	yogurt, sugar (in excess)

APPENDIX F
STIPENDS

Stipends, if given, were of equal amount, regardless of age, degrees, or level of competence and given according to individual needs. It is worth looking at the stipend documents in detail, since they reflect much about the center's values and our continuous efforts to stress that payment should depend mainly on constructive, meaningful, relevant, and altruistic efforts, only secondarily on money.

CRITERIA FOR RECEIVING A STIPEND, I (1971)

Anyone who feels she/he (note our early effort to desexualize the language) has met the criteria listed below should submit a written request for a stipend. The primary considerations are (1) the needs of the Center, and (2) available money.

Since we are now trying to develop a core of full-time "generally" trained persons (generalists) to work at the center, one important criterion is that the person be presently working at Fort Help in a full-time capacity (about thirty hours a week or more), functioning in several areas of the center's work. Although we all specialize in a particular function, e.g., greeting, individual counseling, group work, coordination or training, and have a special interest area(s), e.g., sexuality, overeating, etc., a generalist seeking a stipend should have demonstrated commitment to several functions at the center and have an interest and some knowledge about other program areas than his/her specialty. As with assessing new staff members, we are most interested in individuals whose training is sufficient to be self-directed in their interest area, which includes program coordinators.

Another consideration is long-term commitment. Individuals who have been functioning productively and fairly consistently at the center and have made an indefinite commitment to continue working are given higher priority.

The last consideration is financial need based on minimal living expenses.

STIPEND CRITERIA, II (1972)

1. Minimum twenty hours a week commitment, hopefully more.
2. Making a major contribution to the center.
3. Adherence to Fort Help policies of nondrug use, no smoking in the center, being available to provide immediate help, and becoming a generalist-problem solver.
4. Commitment to the overall goals and philosophy of Fort Help: (a) Helping people of all ages, races, sexes, socioeconomic backgrounds, and religious and political beliefs; (b) Willingness to work or learn to work in the areas we deal with: sex, drugs, obesity, death and dying, suicide, etc.; (c) Making the center self-supporting; (d) Maintaining the ban on violence and drug use in the center; (e) Maintaining the high quality of helping services, in warm, supportive atmosphere, trying not to create unnecessary dependencies of long-term therapy or involvement, or involvement sexually or financially with our guests.

The twenty-hour minimal time commitment is set to assure that the person has enough contact with the daily business of the Center to have a thorough knowledge of its operation. It is better to be at the Center several days a week than to spend several hours in few days at a time.

PROCEDURES FOR GETTING STIPEND

1. A person should make a written request of financial need and the specifications of his/her eligibility: (a) hours per week—and length of commitment to the center (b) statement of contribution to the center (c) statement of willingness to adhere to and agree with Fort Help's general goals and philosophy (d) financial need

2. Request will be reviewed by the core group.

Stipends are allotted in the same amount on a weekly basis according to individual needs and in conjunction with the center's resources and needs.

REQUIREMENTS OF NEW SPACE

We made a careful itemization of reasons for our need for more space. We also organized our actual move by listing and dividing the work among the staff members.

> A gathering place for clients
> Library for staff use
> Group rooms
> Sound proofing
> Kid "corral"
> Carpeting
> Drapes
> Crafts gift shop
> Sleeping room with adjacent shower
> Kitchen
> Telephone crisis room
> Staff lounge

Floor planning

1. What size rooms, and how many of each size? Rooms the size of Peace (rooms were again to be given names to get away from numbers and to convey a positive message - Humanity, Excellence, Joy, Happiness, etc.) have the advantage of being usable for both group and individual work, but too large a room prevents a feeling of intimacy. After long discussion it was decided that we would create between twelve and sixteen soundproof helping/counseling rooms—one-third would be the size of Sunshine, one-third the size of Vibrations (appropriate for four people), one-third the size of Peace. In addition, there would be one large lecture (training) room.

2. "Greeting" area—should it be open and informal, or enclosed? We decided we ought to have a choice. It's nice to talk informally in the open, but if someone is especially upset it would be good to have two or three small rooms adjacent to the greeting area reserved for greeting but usable as overflow for on-going counseling if necessary.

   Should there be telephones in the greeting area? Telephones disrupt "living room" atmosphere, detract attention from guests. We decided to separate greeting from phones, and to begin scheduling *two* staff members at all times, one for phone help, one for greeting.

3. Use of floors. It was generally agreed that we reserve the second floor for quiet counseling space, and that all telephone/office work, greeting, waiting, etc., would be confined to the first floor.

4. Should there be a separate waiting area for the methadone program? Points in favor: This program has heavy traffic every day which will increase when the new federal regulations go into effect. Unlike guests of other programs, methadone guests tend to know one another and to socialize here, which seems to be a therapeutic process for them. A special waiting area would make it possible for them to do this freely without disturbing other guests. Points against: This would segregate one group of guests from others. The question remained unresolved but was to crop up later in our development.

5. Office area. Many questions came up concerning this area. Should telephones be separate from typewriters and conversation? Should there be a separate room for crisis calls or just sound-deadened booths in the corner of the office area? Lothar pointed out that we should plan for staff interaction and companionship as much as for efficiency in working. Even though the present "vault" is noisy, crowded and frustrating, it brings us all together frequently and facilitates communication.

PROGRESS REPORT, SEPTEMBER 1971

ACCOMPLISHMENTS

1. Help, direct and by phone, to thousands in need
2. New organizational concept
3. Model for attack on social problems
4. Involvement
5. Inspiration and hope
6. Living room physical environment
7. New personal and love relationships for numerous staff members

PROBLEMS

1. Human nature: pettiness, hostility, hypocrisy, rumor-mongering, polarization aggravated by ambitious goals, future shock, the often frustrating nature of the very serious and complicated problems we encounter and finding ideal balance between freedom and structure.
2. Money: insufficient donations, contributions, fees from nonheroin clients; unpaid debts of addicts; theft and lack of prevention measures against; insufficient fund raising from foundations and the public.
3. Staff: need more experts in sexual and drug therapy, and more generalists and greeters.
4. Subprograms: delays in alcohol, smoking, sex programs.
5. Smoking and drinking within center.
6. Confidentiality: telephones, written records, traffic around communications area.
7. Greeter malfunctioning.
8. Failure to attract middle-class clientele.

PROPOSED RESTRUCTURING AND TIMETABLE

1. Centralize authority, responsibility, and accountability for heroin program, i.e. reorganize staff, if methadone treatment continues; require one-month payment in advance and each subsequent week in advance for each new guest, payments collected by an independent staff, shift methadone dispensing time to early AM, and move program elsewhere.

2. Phase in complete sex therapy and marital-divorce programs by November 1 (1971).

3. Phase in alcohol program by December 1, smoking by January 1, sleep by March 1, gambling by April 1, death by June 1.

4. Expand space and hours.

5. Formalize telephone counseling.

6. Organize comprehensive training (college) program starting with greeter-generalists, then sex therapy, alcohol, etc., i.e., combine outside experts with in-house personnel.

7. Complete and check on system of individual consultants; post list.

8. Expand small (peer) group concept.

9. Conduct regular open house events.

10. Examine records of past applicants and former staff members; attempt reinvolvement.

11. Carry out ethic on nonsmoking, beginning with leadership group.

REPRESENTATIVE FINANCIAL STATEMENTS OF THE MID-PERIOD

STATEMENT OF REVENUE AND EXPENSES
YEAR ENDING DECEMBER 31, 1974

REVENUE	1st Quarter	2nd Quarter	3rd Quarter	4th Quarter	Total Year
Direct Methadone	8,710.63	7,459.50	6,999.82	9,390.88	32,560.83
Direct Counseling	11,199.89	11,225.09	9,243.71	10,895.84	42,564.53
Medi-Cal Fees	9,108.50	11,887.50	11,150.96	12,127.81	44,274.77
Contributions	3,750.00	3,950.00	4,750.00	—	12,450.00
Miscellaneous	—	830.57	1,014.90	—	1,845.47
Interest Income	—	32.58	38.16	122.48	193.22
Total Revenue	32,769.02	35,385.24	33,197.55	32,537.01	133,888.82
EXPENSES					
Methadone Stipends	9,650.92	9,272.95	9,613.66	9,889.86	38,427.39
Counseling Stipends	10,282.52	12,292.30	13,516.42	13,042.47	49,133.71
Office	1,333.33	1,568.02	2,171.25	2,397.08	7,469.68
Rent & Utilities	2,617.01	1,952.21	2,604.07	2,554.29	9,727.58
Insurance	1,068.37	705.58	1,240.47	828.99	3,843.41
Methadone Program	4,163.14	4,208.90	3,855.17	3,364.86	15,592.07
Maintenance	608.68	1,246.15	1,118.76	255.66	3,229.25
Miscellaneous	2,748.99	3,062.90	1,508.72	1,678.13	8,998.74
TOTAL EXPENSES	32,472.96	34,309.01	35,628.52	34,011.34	136,421.83
EXCESS (DEFICIT) OF REVENUE OVER EXPENSE	296.06	1,076.23	(2,430.97)	(1,474.33)	(2,533.01)

STATEMENT OF REVENUE AND EXPENSES
YEAR ENDING DECEMBER 31, 1975

REVENUE	1st Quarter	2nd Quarter	3rd Quarter	4th Quarter	Total Year
Counseling Fees	13,598.09	13,495.73	11,293.85	12,204.07	50,591.74
Methadone Fees	9,164.95	9,264.14	7,469.00	7,485.09	33,383.18
Medical Fees	20,117.76	13,571.00	20,124.00	20,751.01	74,563.77
Contributions	192.40	1,035.62	—	2,640.00	3,868.02
Interest Income	—	46.17	50.46	68.37	165.00
Miscellaneous	—	395.90	309.12	108.70	813.72
Total Revenue	43,073.20	37,808.56	39,246.43	43,257.24	163,385.43
EXPENSES					
Counseling Stipends	12,130.85	10,903.80	9,217.00	11,435.00	43,686.65
Methadone Stipends	12,214.54	11,118.14	11,552.85	11,405.70	46,291.23
Other Stipend Expense	3,309.33	2,358.64	1,686.51	1,895.86	9,250.34
Office Expense	2,261.98	1,132.37	1,264.83	2,159.43	6,818.61
Rent & Utilities	3,329.13	2,649.41	3,562.25	2,518.23	12,059.02
Insurance	1,248.43	552.66	—	1,812.37	3,613.46
Methadone Program	4,587.79	2,612.42	2,188.49	2,715.15	12,103.85
Maintenance	3,237.76	1,907.38	1,432.07	1,387.75	7,934.96
Operating Expense	1,178.01	1,458.21	1,407.38	1,462.06	5,505.66
Miscellaneous	386.11	62.60	111.91	43.82	601.44
Total Expenses	43,883.93	34,755.63	32,423.29	36,805.37	147,868.22
EXCESS (DEFICIT) OF REVENUE OVER EXPENSE	(810.73)	3,052.93	6,823.14	6,451.87	15,517.21

FORT HELP Combined Statement of Financial Position
December 31, 1978 and 1979

	December 31, 1978		December 31, 1979	
ASSETS:				
Checking, cash				
Counseling	7,131.50		2,778.56	
Methadone	13,509.64		15,738.92	
Savings, counseling	13,781.00		9.72	
Ready Assets, counseling	0		1,110.33	
Total Cash		34,422.14		19,637.53
Accounts Receivable				178.33
Prepaid Insurance		1,400.00		2,656.55
Equipment - Net		0		745.50
Total Assets		35,822.14		23,217.91
LIABILITIES & EQUITY				
Salaries payable	1,480.69		1,882.44	
Accounts payable	0		772.38	
Liabilities		1,480.69		2,654.82
Fund Balances				
Counseling	22,768.32		5,752.63	
Methadone	11,383.92		15,169.07	
Violence line	189.21		(357.61)	
Net Worth		34,341.45		20,563.09
TOTAL LIABILITIES & EQUITY		35,822.14		23,217.91

COMMENTS FROM STAFF MEMBERS

LEADERSHIP

A true leader is a follower—the 97% lead, not the 3%.

I had more gripes about this than any other aspect of the Center, due mostly to the number of leaders. I admired Joel's courage and experimentation and grew to like him. Liking your leader was a good concept to learn in such a depersonalized society as ours.

I respect the way Joel avoids being stuck with all the responsibility and authority.

Rare to find democracy in action! Harder to work in but, I found, much more growth producing than a typical work situation.

Willingness to help everyone, regardless of income.

We do run the place, for better or for worse—it's ours to do with as we feel necessary.

The "alternative" lies in the willingness to struggle, not necessarily in the success or the results."

To me an "alternative" organization is one in which people of different life styles, ages, philosophies, etc., can work together without imposing their personal prejudices on each other—live and let live.

An alternative for the helpers, many of them wouldn't be that unless Fort Help were there.

Collective decisionmaking and flexibility of everything.

WHICH CONCEPTS WOULD YOU USE IN YOUR OWN CENTER?

Be loose (if possible) on credentials, not make it a lucrative therapy center (volunteer concept), and share administrative tasks.

Keep the casualness of the atmosphere for our clients and ourselves; maintain assessment process, consulting functions, intra-staff sociability, freedom of choice about caseloads.

Hire people on the basis of their understanding and acceptance of their humanity and knowledge of the dynamics of human behavior—a combination of both is ideal.

Have a similar setting, definitely keep the nonbureaucratic democratic policy-making procedures, provide the same combination of client experience, staff involvement, and "community" emphasis.

Plunge in (perhaps Joel's greatest contribution)—a belief that most anything can be done. Similar emphasis on staff qualities, i.e., ability over paper credentials. Similar broad appeal: anyone welcome, all kinds of problems, all incomes (flexible scale). Similar linking of therapy and politics that existed for some of us; therapy to help people exist in the world, not how to conform. Similar anti-medical model, etc. Similar respect for people and their ability to say what they want. Similar (in general) emphasis on short-term therapy.

WHAT MADE FORT HELP AN "ALTERNATIVE"

Everybody sharing administrative work, no secretaries, no federal funds, few grants, nonmedical orientation, volunteer concept.

The fact that any staff member can take responsibility for doing or starting anything without waiting for a boss to approve, although he/she may run into the resistance of the entire staff.

Concentrated on change rather than adjustment.

Freedom from outside political control.

Most important aspect is the interchange and development of ideas in a conducive environment.

Providing much more of an opportunity to exercise power in shaping our experience than other institutions.

Allowing for change and group decision.

It's one of the few places inexpensive enough to meet the needs of low income people.

HOW IT AFFECTED PERSONAL LIVES OF STAFF MEMBERS

Gaining self confidence, friends.

An incredible amount: Fort Help is probably the finest growth experience I've ever had.

It taught me about a lifestyle totally different from my own and has been helpful in teaching me to cope with future shock.

Good friendships—one of the important things in life to me.

Involvement in something that had great meaning for me.

Observing Joel's ability to support others in 'doing their own thing'—doing something the way they wanted without needing to control or direct the entire process.

WHY THEY LEFT

Because I became a foster mother to two little girls.

To start San Francisco Sex Information.

Too draining in addition to full-time job.

Weary of being criticized rather than supervised.

Overcommitted in graduate school, paying job and a clinical internship.

Money.

To escape the increasing egalitarianism. I enjoyed being with many capable people but resented being underpaid while people with limited skills received the same compensation.

There was nothing further I felt I could give or get from the Fort at that time.

I had a full-time job and didn't feel I could put in enough time to make a significant contribution or to gain much myself from being there.

Wanted another experience; bored by repetitiveness of staff struggles; wanted to be around more experienced staff.

Experienced a growing irritation at the talk-a-lot, do-nothing people.

Simply time for new experiences. Also, my own need to obtain credentialing which would allow me a greater range of economic or life style alternatives.

GOOD ASPECTS OF FORT HELP

It has brought together a good group of people who are taking care of themselves as an organization with no vested interest.

It actually *exists!* And in spite of all, we have endured through constant struggle, no money, people coming and going, conflicts of philosophy and organization. We actually keep growing, changing and *attempting* to live up to our ideals, including offering services that are very hard to find for low fees.

It has encouraged creativity in its staff instead of the conformity required by more traditional agencies.

Respect for people (usually) and their rights and abilities to deal with their lives. Lack of competition, willingness of co-workers to give and ask for help. Values of most of the staff, their views of society. Attempt to build confidence and independence rather than dependence.

It is imperative that society has alternatives to current agencies. Hopefully places like Fort Help will influence these to become more humanistic and less bureaucratic, meanwhile giving people a place to go where they are not seen as merely sick. Also, provides space for people who are not trained as therapists to receive training at the same time they give help.

Interdisciplinary staff; variety of ways of helping; credible objection to medical model.

A wonderful place to get the idea that needing emotional help doesn't mean you are sick or crazy—and then get help.

Eliminated negative concept of *patients*.

Mostly the concern of the counselors for their clients and their very strong desire to help.

It gave me the feeling of *having* a professional life.

I clarified and experienced first-hand most of what I had learned in books.

I learned about a whole new area of counseling (sexuality) and also got required hours for my license.

Received my master's degree using Fort Help as field work.

It provided contacts which later proved very important in my doctoral research.

It gave me the background needed to recruit volunteers for a rap crisis center.

Led to my decision to go to graduate school.

Fort Help enabled me to follow through on my previous plan to become a professional therapist, and especially to acquire all-round competence rather than just a degree.

HOW DID FORT HELP AFFECT YOUR PROFESSIONAL LIFE?

Started me on a second career.

Changed my life completely. I'd never thought of therapy as a career before."

I enjoy the association with an alternative group—lots of new ideas and a place to try them out or bounce them off others.

Reinforced my antiprofessionalism. . .it did not motivate me to go back to school, nor to get degrees—the opposite, if anything. I learned I could get what I needed and practice therapy without the pieces of paper.

On my vita this experience evokes extremely mixed reactions and provides a barometer of the social consciousness of the people I'm talking with.

It is very rare for a woman under 30 to have the opportunity to know the scope and share the administration of a $200,000 operation. The experience gave me a feeling of efficacy and confidence that carries into almost any kind of work I may do.

HOW DID FORT HELP AFFECT YOUR PERSONAL LIFE?

Would take volumes to explain—primarily gave me hope that change for the better can happen.

As a result of being at Fort Help I became open to a lot of different ideas and lifestyles.

I was depressed and lonely when I came to Fort Help, in a line of work that had outrun its usefulness; today I'm working at something I enjoy. My professional partner, now my wife, came to me out of relationships started at Fort Help.

Fort Help did not change my personal life much since I was not looking for relationships with staff members.

I have always worked in fringe areas and there is a certain feeling of security in knowing others who are also working in frontier areas.

I've grown and changed a great deal, learned more about myself as I learned more about therapy.

SUMMARY OF INFORMATION REGARDING CLIENTS AND SERVICES

Generalizing from Lothar's results on clients' growth or change while coming to Fort Help, we see that apart from telephone help, education, and crisis intervention, those people who were the most motivated to keep working on their problems over a long period of time reaped the greatest rewards. It took exactly one month for fifty greetings to take place, and exactly another month for the next fifty. Our caseload increased dramatically after that, as did the number of people coming in for continuing help.

There were fifty-one men, thirty-six women, ten couples (eight heterosexual, one homosexual males, one homosexual females).

1. Time of first visit: Noon, ten; 1 P.M., ten; 2 P.M., 19; 3 P.M., sixteen; 4 P.M., eleven; 5 P.M., eight; 6 P.M., eight; 7 P.M., three; 8 P.M., three.

2. Residence: San Francisco, sixty-eight; East Bay area, eleven; San Mateo County, six; Sonoma County, three; Santa Clara County, one; no address given, one.

3. Employed: Yes, fifty-six; No, thirty-seven. Many of the employed do not have jobs per se, but do something from which they derive a subsistence income. In terms of state-recognized "work," approximately fifty percent of our people are "unemployed."

4. Age: To 19, two; 20-25, thirty-one; 26-29, eighteen; 30-34, twenty; 35-39, four; 40-44, six; 45-49, two; 50 and over, seven. The youngest was 17 and the oldest 81.

5. Income: None, twenty-seven; $0-199, eleven; $200-399, nine; $400-599, fourteen; $600-799, eight; $800-999, two; $1,000-1,499, eight; $1,500 up, two.

    Approximately half the guests in this sample earned less than $200 a month. We certainly were getting a population that could not afford these services at conventional fee-for-service facilities.

6. Fees: Medi-Cal, seventeen; $0-4, eleven; $5-9, eleven; $10-14, ten; $15-19, five; $20-24, eight; $25-29, one; $30+, one; No fee, thirty-one.

One third of the greetings ended with people not paying for greetings. Our average fee was between $10 and $12. Many people wrote Medi-Cal with a question mark and more fees were listed as Medi-Cal than payment stickers submitted.

They heard about Fort Help from widely scattered sources: friends (twenty-six); radio (twelve, half of whom mentioned Don Chamberlain); Fort Help staff directly (nine); mental health agencies (eight); women's organizations (six); passed by the place (five); *People's Yellow Pages* (a directory of alternative services) (three).

Guest reasons for coming (some areas tended to overlap, such as relationship and sex):

Relationship	27	Body symptoms	2
Deep anxiety	23	Insomnia	1
Sex	21	Drugs	7
Alienation/loneliness	15	Alcohol	7
Relationship break-up	13	Family	6
Homosexuality	12	Suicide	5
"Magic-seeker"	11	Falling apart	4
Poor self-image	9	Feminine oppression	6
Growth	13	Eating	3
Dealing with feelings	9	The blahs	5
Want to be taken care of	2	Dealing with kids	5
Creative blocks	2	Heavy paranoia	2

Remember, this only includes a hundred first-time greetings, not telephone contacts or guests who go directly into groups without greetings, or those coming in for second or subsequent visits.

Lothar did a study of eighty-eight people who came to the center (twenty-four of these were seen one time only, either in an intake capacity, referred, declined or cancelled follow-up appointments and were not scored):

Number seen more than once	64 (72.7%)
Number seen one month or less	13 (14.8%)
Number seen from one to six months	42 (47.7%)
Number seen longer than six months	9 (10.2%)

By age:

Under 25	24 (27.2%)
25 - 40	39 (44.3%)
40 - 55	21 (23.8%)
Over 55	4 (4.5%)

"Growth" results are of course purely subjective, and were scored very cautiously; in case of doubt, the lower rating was given. Among the clients seen once (twenty-four) and those seen for one month or less (thirteen), there were only two cases, one each, of reported positive effects, both involving impotence. Growth was measured at termination, since no follow-up system exists.

However, in addition to these effects of short-term intervention, significant initial growth was experienced by many of the clients who stayed for intermediate or long-term help.

Among clients who were seen for more than six months the only disappointing results were in two cases involving heavy, long-time alcoholism which eventually negated the temporarily achieved growth.

Taking the under-25 group into account as well, it appears that clients under 40 were less likely to get discouraged initially, but had a lower eventual success rate than the 40 to 55 group.

The problem areas (some cases fall into more than one category and therefore the total adds up to more than 100%):

Marriage relationship or sexual	62 (70.4%)
Family unit (parents or children)	15 (17%)
Alcohol and other drugs	11 (12.5%)
Others including depression	32 (36.4%)

SELECTED BIBLIOGRAPHY

Argyris, C., *Integrating the Individual and the Organization*, New York: Wiley, 1964.

Bailey, R. and Brake, M. (eds.), *Radical Social Work*, New York: Pantheon Books, 1975.

Bartlett, L., *New Work/New Life*, New York: Harper & Row, 1976.

Bennis, W. G., *Changing Organizations*, New York: McGraw-Hill, 1966.

Benson, J. (ed.), *Organizational Analysis: Critique and Innovation*, Beverly Hills: Sage Publications, 1977.

Blau, P. and Scott, W., *Formal Organizations*, San Francisco, Chandler Publishing, 1962.

Bloch, A., *Murphy's Law and Other Reasons Why Things Go Wrong*, Los Angeles: Price, Stern, Sloan, 1977.

Bok, S., *Lying*, New York: Pantheon, 1978.

Bolles, R., *What Color Is Your Parachute?*, Berkeley: Ten Speed Press, 1978.

Case, John, and Taylor, R. (eds.), *Co-ops, Communes & Collectives*, New York: Pantheon Books, 1979.

Dale, E., *Management Theory and Practice*, New York: McGraw-Hill, 1965.

DeGrazia, S., *Of Time, Work and Leisure*, New York: Kraus, 1973.

Dickson, P., *The Future File*, New York: Avon, 1977.

Drucker, P., *The Effective Executive*, New York: Harper and Row, 1966.

Dvorin, E., *From Amoral to Humane Bureaucracy*, San Francisco: Canfield, 1972.

Edelwich, J., *Burnout in the Helping Professions*, New York: Human Sciences Press, 1980.

Ellul, J., *The Technological Society*, New York: Knopf, 1964.

Fabun, D., *The Dynamics of Change*, New York: Prentice-Hall, 1967.

Fairfield, R., (ed.), *Utopia, U.S.A.*, San Francisco: Alternative Foundation, 1972.

Fairweather, G., *Methods for Experimental Social Innovation*, New York: Wiley & Sons, 1968.

Festinger, L., *et. al.*, *Social Pressures in Informal Groups*, Stanford: Stanford University Press, 1950.

Flory, C., *Managing Through Insight*, New York: Mentor, 1968.

Fort, J., *Sound Mind, Sound Society*, Berkeley: University of California Extension (Independent Study), 1980.

Fort, J., *The Unreasonable Man*, San Francisco: KQED-TV and PBS, 1970.

Foucault, M., *Madness and Civilization*, New York: Mentor, 1965.

Frank, J., *Persuasion and Healing*, Schocken, 1974.

Fromm, E., *The Anatomy of Human Destructiveness*, New York: Fawcett Books, 1973.

Goffman, E., *The Presentation of Self in Everyday Life*, New York: Anchor, 1959.

Gottesfield, H., [IT]et. al. (eds.), *Strategies in Innovative Human Services*, New York: Behavioral Publications, 1973.

Guerney, B., *Psychotherapeutic Agents: New Roles for Non-Professionals*, New York: Holt, Rinehart & Winston, 1969.

Guttentage, M. (ed.), *Handbook of Evaluation*, Beverly Hills: Sage Publications, 1975.

Hale, A. Paul, *Handbook of Small Group Research*, 2nd ed., New York: The Free Press, 1976.

Haley, J., *Problem Solving Therapy*, San Francisco: Jossey-Bass, 1977.

Harrington, A., *Life in the Crystal Palace*, New York: Knopf, 1959.

Harrop, D., *Paychecks: Who Makes What*, New York: Harper & Row, 1980.

Hatry, H., *Practical Program Evaluation for State and Local Government Officials*, Urban Institute: Washington, D.C., 1973.

Henry, N., *Doing Public Administration*, Boston: Allyn & Bacon, 1978.

Higdon, H., *The Business Healers*, New York: Random House, 1969.

Hirschman, A., *Exit, Voice and Loyalty: Responses to Decline in Firms, Organizations and States*, Cambridge: Harvard University Press, 1970.

Holleb, F., *Alternatives to Community Mental Health*, Boston: Beacon Publishers, 1976.

Holloway, M., *Heavens on Earth: Utopian Communities in America, 1680-1880*, New York: Dover Books, 1966.

Huff, D., *How to Lie with Statistics*, New York: Norton, 1954.

Jay, A., *Corporation Man*, New York: Pocket Books, 1973.

Judgson, A., *A Manager's Guide to Making Changes*, New York: Wiley and Sons, 1966.

Kanter, R., *Commitment and Community: Communes and Utopias in Sociological Perspective*, Cambridge: Harvard University Press, 1972.

Kaplan, H.S., *The New Sex Therapy*, New York: Brunner/Mazel, 1974.

Kaufman, H., *Red Tape*, Brookings Institution: Washington, D.C., 1967.

Kaufman, H., *The Limits of Organizational Change*, Birmingham: University of Alabama Press, 1971.

Kelso, L, and Adler, M., *The Capitalist Manifesto*, New York: Random House, 1958.

Koch, J., & L., *The Marriage Savers*, New York: Coward & McCann, 1976.

Kovel, J., *A Complete Guide to Therapy*, New York: Pantheon Books, 1976.

Lakein, A., *How to Get Control of Your Time and Your Life*, New York: Signet, 1974.

Lambro, D., *The Federal Rathole*, New Rochelle: Arlington House, 1975.

Levinson, H., *Executive Stress*, New York: Harper & Row, 1970.

Likert, R., *New Patterns of Management*, New York: McGraw-Hill, 1961.

Likert, R., *Some Applications of Behavioral Research*, Paris, France: UNESCO, 1967.

Litterer, J. (ed.), *Organizations*, New York: John Wiley, 1969.

Lubove, R., *The Professional Altruist*, New York: Atheneum Publishers, 1969.

Marris, P. & Rein, M., *Dilemmas of Social Reform*, London, England: Penguin Books, 1972.

McGee, R., *Crisis Intervention in the Community*, Baltimore: University Park Press, 1974.

Merton, R., *Leader in Bureaucracy*, New York: Free Press, 1952.

Michels, R., *Political Parties: a Sociological Study of the Oligarchical Tendencies of Modern Democracy*, New York: Dover, 1959.

Mills, C., *The Power Elite*, Oxford, England: Oxford University Press, 1978.

Nakamura, R., and Smallwood, F., *The Politics of Policy Implementation*, New York: St. Martin's Press, 1980.

Negley, G., and Patrick, J., *The Quest for Utopia*, New York: Anchor, 1952.

Nisbet, R., *History of the Idea of Progress*, New York: Basic Books, 1980.

OM Collective, The, *The Organizer's Manual*, New York: Bantam, 1971.

Otto, H. (ed.), *The New Sexuality*, Palo Alto: Science & Behavior Books, 1971.

Parkinson, C., *The Law*, Boston: Houghton-Mifflin, 1980.

Peter, L., and Hull, R., *The Peter Principle*, New York: Morrow, 1969.

Presthus, R., *The Organizational Society*, New York: Vintage, 1965.

Revel, J., *Without Marx or Jesus*, New York: Doubleday, 1971.

Rohrlich, J., *Work and Love*, New York: Summit Books, 1980.

Rosenberg, S., *Self-Analysis of Your Organization*, New York: American Management Assn., 1974.

Sale, K., *Human Scale*, New York: Coward, McCann, 1980.

Sayles, L., *Managing Large Systems*, New York: Harper & Row, 1971.

Schumacher, E., *Small Is Beautiful*, New York: Harper & Row, 1973.

Shafritz, J., and Hyde, A., (eds.), *Classics of Public Administration*, Oak Park, IL: Moore Publishing, 1978

Shepperd, C., *Working in the 21st Century*, New York: Behavioral Science, 1980.

Simon, H., *Administrative Behavior: a Study of Decision-Making Processes in Organization*, New York: Free Press, 1976.

Smith, A., *Powers of Mind*, New York: Random House, 1975.

Sobey, F., *The Non-Professional Revolution in Mental Health*, New York: Columbia University Press, 1970.

Spiegel, D., & P., *Outsiders U.S.A.*, New York: Rinehart, 1973.

Stevens, R., *American Medicine and the Public Interest*, New Haven: Yale University Press, 1971.

Terkel, S., *Working*, New York: Pantheon Books, 1972.

Thomas, H., *The Living World of Philosophy*, Philadelphia: Blakiston, 1946.

Thomas, J., and Bennis, W., *Management of Change and Conflict*, Baltimore: Penguin Books, 1972.

Toffler, A., *Future Shock*, New York: Random House, 1970.

Townsend, R., *Up the Organization*, New York: Knopf, 1970.

VonMises, L., *Bureaucracy*, New York: Arlington House, 1969.

Weber, M., *From Max Weber: Essays in Sociology*, Edited by Gerth & Mills, New York: Oxford University Press, 1946.

Weiss, C., *Evaluation Research*, New Jersey: Prentice-Hall, 1972.

Westin, A., *Privacy and Freedom*, New York: Atheneum, 1967.

Zimbardo, P., *et. al.*, *Influencing Attitudes and Changing Behavior*, San Francisco: Addison-Wesley, 1977.

INDEX

135